Multiple Choice Questions in Pharmacology

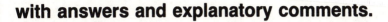

with answers and explanatory comments.

Second edition

A D'Mello MSc, PhD

Former Head and Senior Lecturer, Pharmacology Section
Department of Pharmacology and Therapeutics, The London Hospital
and Medical College.

and

Z L Kruk MSc, PhD

Reader in Neuropharmacology, Department of Pharmacology,
Queen Mary and Westfield College, London.

Edward Arnold
A division of Hodder & Stoughton
LONDON MELBOURNE AUCKLAND

Contents

Introduction

Multiple choice questions (MCQs) are increasingly used in examinations as they allow a wide range of knowledge to be tested and are an objective means of assessing students. There is still an opinion prevalent that MCQs measure only factual recall, and teachers may therefore be interested in attempts made in this book to formulate questions which test knowledge of concepts as opposed to drug names. We have found that such questions can be used to identify learning difficulties encountered by students, whether these be problems of remembering or distinguishing drug names, or difficulties in understanding concepts or conventional terms. For example, Questions 8 and 9 deal with receptors involved in eliciting particular responses in the eye. Questions 10 and 11 are linked with Questions 8 and 9 in that they test knowledge of the same responses, except that the stems of the questions introduce the named drugs. Many of the questions on central nervous system (CNS) pharmacology have a similar design to those on the autonomic nervous system, and they incorporate ideas on the interactions of drugs with receptors.

The questions in the this book have been selected from among those which have been evaluated on preclinical medical students at various stages of their course in pharmacology at The London Hospital Medical College. Some questions appear considerably easier than others; it should be remembered that they would have been presented to students at different stages of their course. The conventional construction of MCQs has been used throughout. A stem is followed by five possible alternatives, any number of which may be true or false and each one of which should be attempted. The correct response with comments appear on the facing page.

The text of the First Edition has been considerably revised. Questions relating to new knowledge on several topics, for example receptors, autacoids and hormones, have been added. The section which includes pharmacokinetics has been extended. Several problem solving questions have been introduced.

We hope that this book will help students to overcome their well-known apprehension of MCQs, and that teachers may be encouraged to use MCQs more frequently to assess learning and understanding not only in formal examinations but also in practical classes and demonstrations. We have used MCQs related to some practical classes, and students have found them more beneficial than lengthy formal laboratory reports.

1 In noradrenergic neurones:
   (a) tyrosine is a precursor of noradrenaline.
   (b) the rate-limiting step in the synthesis of noradrenaline is at tyrosine hydroxylase.
   (c) dopamine is decarboxylated to noradrenaline.
   (d) L-DOPA is converted to dopamine inside the storage vesicle.
   (e) isoprenaline is synthesized from noradrenaline.

2 The neuronal uptake 1 process for noradrenaline:
   (a) is specific for noradrenaline.
   (b) is a passive one.
   (c) is Na^+ dependent.
   (d) renders noradrenaline unavailable for further release.
   (e) is blocked by cocaine.

3 The extraneuronal uptake 2 process for amines:
   (a) is specific for noradrenaline.
   (b) inactivates isoprenaline.
   (c) has a higher threshold than uptake 1 for noradrenaline.
   (d) is saturated by low concentrations of noradrenaline.
   (e) is potentiated by hydrocortisone.

4 Acetylcholine:
   (a) is synthesized by acetylcholinesterase.
   (b) is released only from parasympathetic nerves.
   (c) is inactivated by re-uptake into nerves.
   (d) releases adrenaline from the adrenal medulla.
   (e) is released from sympathetic nerves to the sweat glands.

1 (a) **True** L–Tyrosine $\xrightarrow{\text{tyrosine hydroxylase}}$ L–DOPA $\xrightarrow{\text{DOPA decarboxylase}}$

dopamine $\xrightarrow{\text{dopamine β-hydroxylase}}$ noradrenaline.

(b) **True** Tyrosine hydroxylase (and hence the rate of noradrenaline synthesis) is influenced by:
(i) end-product inhibition by noradrenaline,
(ii) presynaptic receptors
(iii) axonal nerve traffic to terminals.

(c) **False** See (a).

(d) **False** This reaction occurs in the cytoplasm.

(e) **False**

2 (a) **False** Adrenaline, dopamine, 5-HT and tyramine are also taken up, but they do not have the same affinity for uptake 1 as noradrenaline does.

(b) **False** It is a high-affinity, low-capacity active uptake process which is saturable.

(c) **True** Na^+ is essential to activate an ATPase which provides the driving force for the uptake pump.

(d) **False** Much of the noradrenaline taken up is stored in vesicles and is available for release by nerve impulses; any noradrenaline not taken up into vesicles is deaminated by MAO.

(e) **True** Drugs that block uptake 1 delay the inactivation of noradrenaline and potentiate it. Other inhibitors of uptake 1 include antidepressants (e.g. imipramine, desipramine, amitriptyline) and amphetamines.

3 (a) **False** It is an uptake process into non-neuronal cells for noradrenaline, dopamine, 5-HT, adrenaline and isoprenaline. Uptake 2 removes high extracellular concentrations of monoamines from the systemic circulation following release of adrenaline and noradrenaline from the adrenal medulla after sympathetic stimulation.

(b) **True** See (a).

(c) **True** It is a lower affinity high capacity system.

(d) **False** It is saturated only by very high concentrations of noradrenaline.

(e) **False** Hydrocortisone and some other steroids block uptake 2; specific or selective inhibitors of uptake 2 are not available.

4 (a) **False** Acetylcholinesterase inactivates acetylcholine.

(b) **False** It is also released:
(i) from postganglionic sympathetic nerves to sweat glands,
(ii) from preganglionic nerves to all autonomic ganglia,
(iii) in the CNS,
(iv) from voluntary nerves to skeletal muscle.

(c) **False** It is inactivated enzymatically:

acetylcholine $\xrightarrow{\text{acetylcholinesterase}}$ choline + acetate.

(d) **True** It acts at nicotinic receptors at this site.

(e) **True** See (b) above.

5 The release of endothelium derived relaxing factor (EDRF):
  (a) can be caused by acetylcholine.
  (b) can be caused by histamine.
  (c) can be prevented by serotonin (5-HT)
  (d) leads to vasodilatation.
  (e) increases availability of Ca^{2+}.

6 Blockade of nicotinic receptors in autonomic ganglia is likely to:
  (a) increase salivary secretion.
  (b) reduce diastolic blood pressure.
  (c) reduce intestinal contractions.
  (d) paralyse striated respiratory muscles.
  (e) cause blurring of vision.

7 Blockade of α_1-adrenoceptors:
  (a) prevents an increase in heart rate due to sympathetic stimulation.
  (b) causes a fall in blood pressure.
  (c) can lead to orthostatic hypotension.
  (d) can cause nasal 'stuffiness'.
  (e) is caused by propranolol.

5 (a) **True** EDRF is believed to be nitric oxide (NO), a molecule synthesized from the amino acid arginine by the actions of arginine oxidases. NO activates soluble guanylate cyclase which catalyzes the conversion of GTP to cyclic GMP. Cyclic GMP decreases the affinity of a calcium-binding protein for calcium (thus decreasing free Ca^{2+}), and so reduces the constrictor tone of vascular smooth muscle.

(b) **True** Not only muscarinic cholinoceptors are involved in the release of EDRF.

(c) **False** Serotonin can release EDRF from coronary arteries which then has a negative modulating role on the vasoconstrictor effect of serotonin. In the absence of endothelium, serotonin exerts a more powerful vasoconstrictor effect.

(d) **True** See (a).

(e) **False** See (a).

6 (a) **False** Salivary secretion is decreased by ganglion blockers (hexamethonium, mecamylamine, pempidine) acting at parasympathetic ganglia. Ganglion blockers are *not* selective for sympathetic or parasympathetic ganglia.

(b) **True** This is an effect due to blockade of sympathetic ganglia.

(c) **True** An action at parasympathetic ganglia.

(d) **False** Skeletal muscle innervation is separate from the autonomic nervous system.

(e) **True** An action at parasympathetic ganglia to the ciliary muscles and iris.

7 (a) **False** An increase in heart rate is mediated by activation of β_1-adrenoceptors.

(b) Sympathetic vasoconstrictor tone is mediated by α_1-adrenoceptors.

(c) **True** The baroreceptor reflex cannot operate because the α_1 (-) adrenoceptors in resistance arterioles are blocked and therefore vasoconstriction cannot occur.

(d) **True** Vasoconstriction (by α-adrenoceptor agonists) in the nasal mucosa causes decongestion.

(e) **False** Propranolol is a β-adrenoceptor blocker. Examples of α-adrenoceptor blockers include prazosin, phentolamine and phenoxybenzamine.

8 Excitation of α-adrenoceptors:
  (a) contracts the radial smooth muscle fibres in the iris.
  (b) contracts the circular smooth muscle fibres in the ciliary muscle.
  (c) retracts the upper eyelid.
  (d) causes vasoconstriction of conjunctival blood vessels.
  (e) causes dilatation of the pupil.   .

9 Excitation of muscarinic receptors:
  (a) contracts the radial smooth muscle fibres in the iris.
  (b) contracts the circular smooth muscle fibres in the ciliary muscle.
  (c) retracts the upper eyelid.
  (d) can cause vasodilatation of conjunctival blood vessels.
  (e) is a mechanism whereby the pupil constricts in bright light.

10 Phenylephrine eye drops:
  (a) constrict the pupil.   .
  (b) move the near point for accommodation nearer.
  (c) retract the upper eyelid.
  (d) cause vasodilatation of conjunctival blood vessels.
  (e) may prevent the pupil from dilating in dull light. .   .

11 Pilocarpine eye drops:
  (a) constrict the pupil.   .
  (b) move the near point for accommodation further away.
  (c) retract the upper eyelid.
  (d) cause vasoconstriction of conjunctival blood vessels.
  (e) may prevent the pupil from dilating in dull light.

	(a)	(b)	(c)	(d)	(e)
8	**True**	**False**	**True**	**True**	**True**
9	**False**	**True**	**False**	**True**	**True**
10	**False**	**False**	**True**	**False**	**False**
11	**True**	**False**	**False**	**False**	**True**

		Innervation	Receptor	Response
Iris	Radial smooth muscle	Sympathetic adrenergic	α-adrenoceptor	Contraction of radial muscle and dilatation of pupil
	Circular smooth muscle	Parasympathetic cholinergic	Muscarinic	Contraction of circular muscle and constriction of pupil
Ciliary body	Circular smooth muscle	Parasympathetic cholinergic	Muscarinic	Contraction of ciliary muscle resulting in less tension on the lens which becomes more spherical. The near point for accommodation moves nearer.
Upper eyelid	Smooth muscle of palpebrae superioris	Sympathetic adrenergic	α-adrenoceptor	Contraction leads to retraction of upper eyelid
Blood vessels of conjunctiva	Circular smooth muscle	Sympathetic adrenergic	α-adrenoceptor	Vasoconstriction, blanching of conjunctiva.
	Smooth muscle		Muscarinic	Vasodilatation, conjunctiva appears red (bloodshot).

Pilocarpine is a muscuarinic receptor agonist.
Phenylephrine is an α-adrenoceptor agonist.

12 If phenylephrine is applied to one eye and tropicamide to the other eye of a human subject:
   (a) both pupils dilate.
   (b) only phenylephrine would abolish the corneal or 'blink' reflex.
   (c) both drugs would move the near point for accommodation nearer the eye.
   (d) both drugs would cause vasodilatation of conjunctival blood vessels.
   (e) only tropicamide would reduce pupillary constriction in bright light.

13 Blockade of β-adrenoceptors:
   (a) results in an increase in heart rate.
   (b) results in a rise in blood pressure.
   (c) prevents the effect of noradrenaline on the isolated heart.
   (d) causes vasodilatation in skeletal muscle.
   (e) is caused by phentolamine.

14 Which of the following statements about β-adrenoceptor blockers are correct?
   (a) lipophilic β-blockers are less likely to cause nightmares than hydrophylic β-blockers.
   (b) hydrophilic β-blockers might accumulate in renal impairment.
   (c) cardioselective β-blockers have no effect on airways resistance.
   (d) non-selective β-blockers can cause coldness of the extremities.
   (e) β-blockers are drugs of choice in treating phaeochromocytoma.

12 (a) **True**   Phenylephrine is an α-adrenoceptor agonist which will cause constriction of the radial muscles of the pupil leading to dilatation; tropicamide is a short-acting muscarinic antagonist which prevents pupillary constriction under the influence of the parasympathetic system. Parasympathetic tone is necessary to maintain normal light-reflex-mediated constriction of the pupil, and if this system is rendered inoperative by a competitive antagonist pupillary dilation will occur.

   (b) **False**   The corneal or blink reflex is mediated by sensory nerves and is independent of the autonomic nervous system.

   (c) **False**   Accommodation for near vision is achieved by stimulation of parasympathetic nerves to circular ciliary muscles, thereby making the lens more spherical. Phenylephrine will have no effect on the near point of vision because there are no α-adrenoceptors in the ciliary muscle; tropicamide will render the near point for vision further away by blocking muscarinic receptors and reducing the circular ciliary muscle tone so that the lens become less spherical.

   (d) **False**   Phenylephrine causes vasoconstriction by action at α_1-adrenoceptors; tropicamide would generally have no effect.

   (e) **False**   Phenylephrine effectively increases sympathetic tone (thus decreasing parasympathetic tone) while tropicamide decreases parasympathetic tone directly. The light reflex operates by virtue of the autonomic nervous system, therefore both drugs could be expected to reduce pupillary constriction in bright light.

13 (a) **False**   β-adrenoceptor agonists cause an increase in force and rate of constriction of the heart.

   (b) **False**   β-adrenoceptor blockers are used as antihypertensives.

   (c) **True**   In the heart, noradrenaline acts at β_1-adrenoceptors.

   (d) **False**   Stimulation of β_2-adrenoceptors in skeletal muscle leads to vasodilatation.

   (e) **False**   Phentolamine is a α-adrenoceptor blocker. Propranolol, oxprenolol and sotalol are β-adrenoceptor blockers.

14 (a) **False**   Lipophilic β-blockers, for example propranolol, are more likely to enter the brain and cause nightmares.

   (b) **True**   Hydrophilic β-blockers, such an atenolol and sotalol, are less subect to liver metabolism than lipophilic β-blockers, and are excreted unchanged by the kidneys; their half-lives are prolonged in renal failure.

   (c) **False**   Such drugs are not cardiospecific. They have less effect on β_2 (bronchial) than β_1-adrenoceptors but can cause bronchospasm in patients with asthma or a history of obstructive airways disease.

   (d) **True**   They do this by blocking β-adrenoceptor mediated vasodilatation in hands and feet.

   (e) **False**   They can be used to control the raised pulse rate in phaeochromocytoma together with an α-adrenoceptor blocker, but never alone, as β-blockers could cause a hypertensive crisis in such a situation because they block β-adrenoceptor mediated vasodilatation (see (d) above).

15 β-adrenoceptor blockers have the following properties:
   (a) oxprenolol has intrinsic sympathomimetic activity.
   (b) when used as antihypertensives, β-blockers often cause orthostatic hypotension.
   (c) propranolol can reduce skeletal muscle tremor in thyrotoxicosis.
   (d) propranolol is used in the treatment of angina.
   (e) they can cause heart block in susceptible individuals.

16 Eye-drops of a drug X cause vasoconstriction of conjunctival blood vessels, contract the radial smooth muscle fibres in the iris, but have no effect on the circular smooth muscle fibres in the ciliary muscle. A drug with such a profile of activity is likely to be:
   (a) a drug for preventing the re-uptake of noradrenaline.
   (b) cocaine.
   (c) phenylephrine.
   (d) a β-adrenoceptor agonist.
   (e) a drug causing blockade of autonomic ganglia.

17 A drug reduces arterial blood pressure, contracts isolated rabbit intestine and increases salivary secretion. To cause all three effects the drug could be:
   (a) a muscarinic receptor agonist.
   (b) a ganglion blocking agent.
   (c) an α-adrenoceptor agonist.
   (d) an α-adrenoceptor antagonist.
   (e) a β-adrenoceptor agonist.

15 (a) **True** Alprenolol, oxprenolol, pindolol and practolol are partial agonists, and are said to have intrinsic sympathomimetic activity (ISA).

(b) **False** This is less likely to occur with β-blockers than with other antihypertensive drugs such as adrenergic neurone blocking agents, probably because reflex vasoconstriction is still possible.

(c) **True** β-adrenoceptor agonists cause tremor by actions on skeletal muscle cells. Tremor caused by the release of adrenaline in thyrotoxicosis can be reduced by propranolol.

(d) **True** β-adrenoceptor blockers reduce the frequency of anginal attacks by decreasing cardiac stimulation provoked by exercise and anxiety.

(e) **True**

16 (a) **True**
   (b) **True**
   (c) **True**
   (d) **False**
   (e) **False** Vasoconstriction of conjunctival blood vessels and contraction of the radial smooth muscle of the iris are caused by activation of α_1-adrenoceptors. There are no alpha-adrenoceptors in the circular smooth muscle fibres in the ciliary muscle. Sympathetic tone maintains a basal release of noradrenaline; thus answers a and b are correct because cocaine is an inhibitor of noradrenaline reuptake and any drug which prolongs the duration of action of noradrenaline might have these effects. Phenylephrine is an α_1-adrenoceptor agonist. A β-adrenoceptor agonist might cause dilatation of conjunctival blood vessels by direct action on β-adrenoceptors on these blood vessels, and a ganglion blocker might be expected to have a similar effect if it were to remove sympathetic vasoconstrictor tone from these blood vessels.

17 (a) **True** Whereas there is no parasympathetic nerve supply to arterial blood vessels, many blood vessels have vestigial muscarinic receptors which can cause vasodilatation when activated by a muscarinic receptor agonist. Muscarinic receptor activation increases intestinal motility and facilitates salivation.

(b) **False** Ganglion blockers will reduce arterial blood presure by inhibiting sympathetic tone; but they will not increase the contraction of isolated rabbit intestine, and they will reduce salivary secretion by blocking parasympathetic ganglia.

(c) **False** An α-adrenoceptor agonist would cause arteriolar constriction and lead to a rise in arterial blood pressure.

(d) **False** An α-adrenoceptor antagonist will not cause contraction of of isolated rabbit intestine or increased salivary secretion.

(e) **False** The same reasoning applies as in (d) above.

18 When given to man a drug causes bradycardia, increased gut motility and pupillary constriction. Which of the following drugs produce this combination of effects?
   (a) adrenaline.
   (b) (+) – tubocurarine.
   (c) acetylcholine.
   (d) noradrenaline.
   (e) neostigmine.

19 β-adrenoceptor blocking compounds may lower blood pressure by the following mechanisms:
   (a) decreasing sympathetically mediated renin release.
   (b) causing vasodilatation in skeletal muscle.
   (c) actions in the CNS.
   (d) decreasing noradrenaline release from sympathetic nerve endings.
   (e) reduction of circulating fluid volume.

20 Salbutamol:
   (a) is devoid of any action on the heart rate.
   (b) contracts uterine smooth muscle.
   (c) causes bronchodilatation.
   (d) can cause skeletal muscle tremor.
   (e) is effective when swallowed.

21 Reserpine:
   (a) prevents the active re-uptake (uptake 1) of noradrenaline from the synaptic cleft into noradrenergic neurones.
   (b) disrupts the storage of monoamines.
   (c) prevents the uptake of noradrenaline from the cytoplasm into noradrenergic storage vesicles.
   (d) has a selective action on noradrenergic neurones only.
   (e) can be used in the treatment of hypertension.

18 (a) **False**   Adrenaline causes initial speeding of the heart, a decrease in gut motility and pupillary dilatation by action on β-adrenoceptors (heart) α and β-adrenoceptors (gut) and α-adrenoceptors (pupil).

  (b) **False**   (+)-tubocurarine works at nicotinic receptors on skeletal muscle and will have little or no effect on any of the systems described at therapeutic concentrations.

  (c) **True**   Acetylcholine acting at muscarinic receptors will cause slowing of the heart, an increase in gut motility and constriction of the circular muscles of the pupil. All these effects mimic the effects of parasympathetic stimulation.

  (d) **False**   Noradrenaline mimics the effects of sympathetic stimulation and all the effects would be the opposite of those described.

  (e) **True**   Neostigmine is an inhibitor of acetylcholinesterase; this leads to a build up of acetylcholine at all parasympathetic junctions, so the reasoning in (c) above applies equally in this case.

19 (a) **True**   Renal sympathetic nerve stimulation or injection of β-adrenoceptor agonists causes renin secretion from the kidney.

  (b) **False**   β-andrenoceptor agonists cause vasodilatation in skeletal muscle. Blockade of β-adrenoceptor mediated vasodilatation may produce pain, cramps and weakness of the muscle when walking.

  (c) **True**   There is evidence that some β-blockers lower blood pressure in animals when injected into the cerebral ventricles and that they antagonize a central pressor action of isoprenaline.

  (d) **True**   Stimulation of presynaptic α-adrenoceptors leads to a decrease of noradrenaline release, whereas stimulation of presynaptic β-adrenoceptors can result in an increased noradrenaline release. Hence β-adrenoceptor blockers may lower blood pressure by this among other mechanisms.

  (e) **True**   This is partly due to the blockade of β-adrenoceptors involved in the release of renin.

20 (a) **False**   Salbutamol selectively activates β_2-adrenoceptors in the bronchioles, especially if it is given by inhalation from an aerosol. If high doses are used, then cardiac stimulation can occur.

  (b) **False**   Uterine smooth muscle is relaxed by β_2-adrenoceptor agonists. Salbutamol is used to prevent premature labour.

  (c) **True**   This is the major use of salbutamol in asthma.

  (d) **True**

  (e) **True**   But usually it is given by inhalation.

21 (a) **False**

  (b) **True**

  (c) **True**   Reserpine and tetrabenazine prevent the active uptake of noradrenaline into the storage vesicles. Reserpine chelates Mg^{2+}, which is necessary for the ATPase which energizes the active transport process. The Mg^{2+} is also needed to stabilize the noradrenaline storage complex. If the Mg^{2+} is chelated, then storage is disrupted.

  (d) **False**   Storage of other monamines, dopamine, 5-HT and adrenaline, is also affected.

  (e) **True**   Depression and drug-induced parkinsonism limit its usefulness.

22 Guanethidine:
  (a) results in decreased release of noradrenaline from noradrenergic nerves in response to sympathetic nerve stimulation.
  (b) can result in the release of noradrenaline.
  (c) can be reversed by indirectly acting sympathomimetic amines.
  (d) can be enhanced by a drug preventing the re-uptake of noradrenaline.
  (e) is used to elevate low blood pressure.

23 Diazoxide.
  (a) is a thiazide.
  (b) is used as a diuretic.
  (c) raises blood sugar.
  (d) dilates arterioles.
  (e) must not be injected intravenously.

24 Nifedipine:
  (a) is a calcium slow-channel agonist.
  (b) increases the flow of Ca^{2+} into cardiac muscle cells.
  (c) reduces left ventricular work.
  (d) relaxes arterial smooth muscle.
  (e) has useful antidysrhythmic activity.

22 (a) **True**   Guanethidine is an adrenergic neurone blocker which decreases noradrenaline release from sympathetic nerves. The exact mechanism is obscure, but a local anaesthetic action has been suggested. Other adrenergic neuron blockers include debrisoquine, bethanidine and bretylium.

    (b) **True**   A transient sympathomimetic action can occur if guanethidine is given intravenously.

    (c) **True**   These appear to displace the adrenergic neurone blocker from the nerve terminal, and then exert their amine releasing effect.

    (d) **False**   Re-uptake blockers (e.g. tricylic antidepressants such as imipramine and amitriptyline) prevent an adrenergic neurone blocker from entering the nerve terminal.

    (e) **False**   Whereas a transient rise in blood pressure may occur – see (b) – adrenergic neurone blockers are used to lower elevated blood pressure.

23 (a) **True**

    (b) **False**   Diazoxide is not a diuretic. It causes salt and water retention.

    (c) **True**   Diazoxide causes hyperglycaemia by inhibiting the release of stored insulin from pancreatic β-cells. It is used orally to treat chronic hypoglycaemia.

    (d) **True**   Diazoxide is a potent vasodilator and antihypertensive drug.

    (e) **False**   Diazoxide is used to obtain immediate control of severe hypertension by intravenous injection. It is unsuitable for long-term oral use in hypertension – see (b) + (c).

24 (a) **False**   Nifedipine is a calcium slow-channel blocking drug which inhibits the entry of Ca^{2+} into cardiac and smooth muscle cells. Nifedipine is believed to increase the frequency of closure of the Ca^{2+} channels.

    (b) **False**   See (a).

    (c) **True**   Nifedipine relaxes smooth muscle and dilates coronary and peripheral arteries so reducing left ventricular work.

    (d) **True**   See (c) and (a).

    (e) **False**   Whilst verapamil has this effect, nifedipine has negligible effects on the cardiac conducting system and so has no useful antidysrhythmic activity.

25 Stimulation of presynaptic α_2-adrenoceptors:
   (a) increases re-uptake of noradrenaline.
   (b) causes vasoconstriction.
   (c) is caused by phentolamine.
   (d) occurs after administration of prazosin.
   (e) occurs after administration of clonidine.

26 At the skeletal neuromuscular junction:
   (a) (+) – tubocurarine is a competitive nicotinic receptor blocker.
   (b) in therapeutic doses, (+) – tubocurarine has a longer duration of action than suxamethonium.
   (c) the actions of (+) – tubocurarine cannot be reversed by neostigmine.
   (d) acetylcholine synthesis and release are impaired in myasthenia gravis.
   (e) pancuronium and gallamine act as desensitization blockers.

27 Suxamethonium:
   (a) is metabolized by plasma cholinesterases.
   (b) can have its neuromuscular blocking effects reversed by anticholinesterases.
   (c) causes depolarization at the endplate.
   (d) does not cause histamine release.
   (e) can cause blockade of nicotinic receptors at ganglia.

25 (a) **False** α_2-adrenoceptors are situated on sympathetic nerve endings (prejunctional α_2-adrenoceptors). If stimulated they reduce the release of noradrenaline. (There are also postjunctional α_2-adrenoceptors).

   (b) **False** See (a).

   (c) **False** Phentolamine is a competitive blocker at postsynaptic α_1- and presynaptic α_2-adrenoceptors. At α_2-adrenoceptors it will tend to enhance neural release of noradrenaline (a major contributory mechanism to the tachycardia caused by phentolamine).

   (d) **False** Prazosin is a highly selective α_1-adrenoceptor blocking agent with little effect on α_2-adrenoceptors. There is relatively little tachycardia caused by prazosin compared to phentolamine.

   (e) **True** This results in a reduction of neuronally released noradrenaline and is presumably partly responsible for the hypotensive action of clonidine.

26 (a) **True** It completes with acetylcholine for the nicotinic receptors on the endplate. There may also be some blockade of nicotinic receptors in ganglia resulting in transient hypotension.

   (b) **True** The relatively brief duration of action of suxamethonium is due largely to its rapid hydrolysis by the pseudocholinesterases of liver and plasma. The action of tubocurarine declines as it is redistributed throughout the extracellular fluid, and most of it is excreted in the urine unchanged.

   (c) **False** The anticholinesterase neostigmine prevents the metabolism of acetylcholine. As the concentration of acetylcholine at the nicotinic receptor rises, it is able to reverse the action of tubocurarine.

   (d) **False** Myasthenia gravis appears to be an autoimmune response in which antibodies are produced to the nicotinic receptors in skeletal muscle.

   (e) **False** They are competitive antagonists at nicotinic receptors on the endplate.

27 (a) **True**

   (b) **False** Anticholinesterases will prevent the metabolism of acetylcholine and suxamethonium and so the depolarization (desensitization) block will be reinforced.

   (c) **True** Suxamethonium has a nicotine-like action at the receptors on the endplate, causing some contractures of the muscle before the block is evident.

   (d) **False** It does release histamine, though to a lesser extent than tubocurarine.

   (e) **True** This may result in transient bradycardia and hypotension, though it should be remembered that suxamethonium is more selective for nicotinic receptors at the endplate than at the ganglia.

28 Hyoscine:
   (a) is a competitive antagonist at muscarinic receptors.
   (b) increases salivary secretion.
   (c) has a short duration of action when applied to the eye.
   (d) causes drowsiness and sedation.
   (e) is used to prevent motion sickness.

29 Which of the following statements about anticholinesterases are correct?
   (a) anticholinesterases can reverse the effects of (+) – tubocurarine.
   (b) DFP (dyflos) is a short acting anticholinesterase.
   (c) in overdose they can cause death by respiratory failure.
   (d) they can decrease intraocular pressure.
   (e) they are used in the diagnosis and treatment of myasthenia gravis.

30 Tyramine:
   (a) is an indirectly acting sympathomimetic amine.
   (b) releases noradrenaline from sympathetic nerve endings.
   (c) is potentiated by monoamine oxidase (MAO) inhibitors.
   (d) is potentiated by uptake inhibitors.
   (e) can cause hypertension in persons treated with monoamine oxidase inhibitors.

28 (a) **True**
   (b) **False** Activation of muscarinic receptors causes salivation.
   (c) **False** Hyoscine causes mydriasis and cycloplegia from which the eye may not fully recover for several days. A much shorter duration of action (several hours) is obtained with tropicamide.
   (d) **True**
   (e) **True**

29 (a) **True** See 26 (c).
   (b) **False** DFP (di-isopropylfluorophosphonate) is an organophosphorus anticholinesterase which inactivates the cholinesterases irreversibly so that recovery depends on formation of fresh enzyme and will take weeks.
   (c) **True** Pulmonary oedema (by excessive bronchial secretions), bronchoconstriction, depression of the respiratory centre, and neuromuscular block of the respiratory muscles (a depolarizing block due to excess acetylcholine) all contribute to respiratory failure.
   (d) **True** When applied to the conjunctiva, anticholinesterases cause constriction of the iris (miosis) and of the ciliary muscle. In some types of glaucoma this may relieve obstruction of the canal of Schlemm, through which aqueous humour drains, and so the intraocular pressure may fall.
   (e) **True** Anticholinesterasses increase the concentration of acetylcholine at the endplate and so render it more effective and improve muscle function in myasthenia gravis.

30 (a) **True** Tyramine enters nerve terminals and releases noradrenaline on to adrenoceptors.
   (b) **True**
   (c) **True** Tyramine is a substrate of monoamine oxidase. See (e).
   (d) **False** Tyramine enters the nerve terminal by the uptake 1 mechanism. Therefore an uptake 1 inhibitor will prevent entry of tyramine into the nerve terminal and so prevent its action.
   (e) **True** Tyramine ingested in food (e.g. some cheeses, chianti) is metabolized by monoamine oxidase in the intestinal wall and liver (first-pass metabolism) so effectively that no systemic effects occur. Inhibition of the monoamine oxidase can result in hypertension if tyramine is ingested.

31 The apparent volume of distribution of a drug:
   (a) is the volume in which a drug is distributed immediately after it is swallowed.
   (b) is the product of the amount of drug in the body and its initial concentration (Co).
   (c) of ethanol would be similar to the volume of total body water.
   (d) of a quaternary ammonium compound would be similar to the volume of extracellular fluid.
   (e) of dextran would be similar to the blood volume.

32 First order kinetics:
   (a) means rate of reaction is proportional to concentration.
   (b) are more common than zero order kinetics.
   (c) apply to exponential processes.
   (d) generally apply to high plasma concentrations (>20 mg/100 ml) of ethanol.
   (e) result in steady-state concentrations after multiple dosing.

31 (a) **False** The apparent volume of distribution of a drug is the volume which would be occupied by a drug if it were present at the same concentration as found in the plasma after intravenous administration. To calculate the apparent volume of distribution (VD) the log plasma concentration of the drug is plotted against time, and this gives a straight line which is extrapolated back to zero time. This plasma concentration at the moment the drug was injected is called C_0 (the concentration at time 0). VD is now calculated from the relationship.

VD = dose $\div$ C_0

The units of VD are litres. For example if 200 mg of drug are given intravenously and C_0 is calculated (after measurements) to be 2 mg per litre, then VD = 200/2 = 100 litres.

(b) **False** See (a).

(c) **True** Ethanol is lipid soluble, and will cross all membranes and distribute throughout the total body water.

(d) **True** A quaternary ammonium compound like tubocurarine is highly ionized and not lipid soluble, and therefore will not cross membranes and will be distributed in extracellular fluid.

(e) **True** Dextran is a mucopolysacharide which is used as a plasma substitute to maintain blood volume in shock.

32 (a) **True** Zero, first and possibly higher orders of kinetics apply to the rates of absorption, metabolism and elimination of drugs. Zero order kinetics, which are not very common in pharmacology, proceed at a *constant rate* and occur when processes are saturated, e.g. high concentrations of ethanol saturating its metabolic enzymes. With first order kinetics the *rate* is directly *proportional to concentration*, i.e. as the concentration falls so does the rate. The equation describing the first order reaction kinetics is rate = kC^n, where C = concentration of reactant, k = the rate constant, and n = 1, the order of reaction. Integration of this equation gives $C = C_0 e^{-kt}$ where C_0 = initial concentration. This is an exponential equation and that is why the term exponential is applied to first order reaction kinetics.

(b) **True** See (a).

(c) **True** See (a).

(d) **False** At plasma concentrations of ethanol greater than 20 mgl/100 ml the enzymes are saturated and zero order kinetics apply. This may not apply to alcoholics in whom enzyme induction may result in first order kinetics even at these higher concentrations. Generally, first order kinetics apply to plasma concentrations of ethanol less *than 10 mg/ml*.

(e) **True** Providing a constant dose is given at equal intervals, then the trough, peak and mean plasma concentrations within a dose interval will approach constant values, i.e. steady state. This is because with first order kinetics the rate of elimination is proportional to the amount of drug in the body. A steady-state concentration occurs when the amount of drug eliminated in the dose interval is the same as the dose given.

33 An ED50:
    (a) is half the dose of a drug producing a maximal contraction of isolated tissue.
    (b) is a measure of antagonism.
    (c) relates to a quantal response produced in 50 per cent of animals.
    (d) is derived in the same way as an LD50
    (e) is used to calculate the therapeutic index.

34 A drug showing first order elimination kinetics from a one-compartment model has a half-time of 6 hours. This means that:
    (a) after 100 mg i.v. 50 mg will be eliminated in 6 hours.
    (b) after 100 mg i.v. 25 mg will be eliminated in 3 hours.
    (c) after 100 mg i.v. 75 mg will be eliminated in 12 hours.
    (d) after 100 mg oral 50 mg will be eliminated in 6 hours.
    (e) after 50 mg i.v. the plasma concentration will fall to 1/8 original concentration after 18 hours.

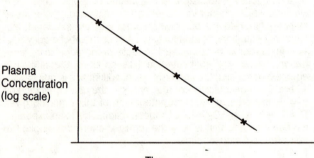

Plasma
Concentration
(log scale)

                              Time

35 In the figure above
    (a) the data describe a single-compartment pharmacokinetic model.
    (b) the data indicate a first order rate process.
    (c) the data indicate an exponential process.
    (d) the slope of the line is numerically equal to first order rate constant.
    (e) the kinetics can be described in terms of a half-time.

33 (a) **False** The term ED50 (ED = Effective Dose) relates to a quantal not a graded response. Quantal responses are measures of a proportion of a population of subjects which reach a criterion response at a given dose of drug. Graded responses are measured on individuals or isolated tissues.

(b) **False** A pAx is a measure of antagonism.

(c) **True** An ED50 is the effective dose in 50 per cent of animals in a group. The response is not death but some other quantal response.

(d) **True** The response in an LD50 (LD = Lethal Dose) is death.

(e) **True** The therapeutic index is the ratio LD50/ED50, and relates only to animal data. The concept of the therapeutic index was originally introduced as the maximum tolerated dose divided by the minimum curative dose to give an idea of the safety of a drug.

34 (a) **True**

(b) **False** In a first order reaction the rate of elimination is proportional to concentration, so that initial rates are higher than those at later times. The *proportion* eliminated *but not the amount* is constant in any given time interval. The time for the initial concentration to fall by a half (t/2) is independent of the initial concentration and is related to the elimination constant by $t/2 = \ln 2/k^*$. The amount remaining at 3 hours is given by $C_0 e^{-kt}$. The elimination rate constant $k = 0.693/6 = 0.116$.

$$100 \times e^{-0.116 \times 3} = 70.7$$

Therefore the amount eliminated is 29.3 mg.

(c) **True** Half is lost in the first 6 hours and half the remainder is lost in the next 6 hours, i.e. ½ 100 + ½ 50 = 75.

(d) **False** For 50 mg to be eliminated within 6 hours. 100 mg must be in the compartment at time 0 (see (a)). However, this will not be the case with oral administration because delayed and possibly incomplete absorption will prevent this.

(e) **True** 18 hours is three half-times, i.e ½ × 1, ½ × ½, ½ × ¼ = ⅛.

35 (a) **True** Note that the Y axis is in log units. As the plasma concentration against time line is straight on this semi logarithmic plot, it means that a single exponential term describes the decreasing plasma concentration of the drug. The data therefore describes a single-compartment model.

(b) **True** The rate of elimination is proportional to concentration, therefore this is a first order rate process.

(c) **True** See a.

(d) **True** The slope of the line $= -K$ (where K is the rate constant).

(e) **True** The half-time is the time taken for the concentration to decline to half of the initial value. This is particularly useful for first order models as it is constant throughout the time when plasma concentrations are measured.

$^*\ln$ = natural log.

36 Single-compartment model means that:
   (a) one exponential term describes the decreasing plasma concentration of the drug.
   (b) a single exponential term describes the rise in plasma concentration following oral administration.
   (c) the drug does not penetrate tissues.
   (d) the drug is restricted to the extracellular fluid.
   (e) the drug is highly ionized.

37 Bioavailability is:
   (a) the difference between the amount of drug absorbed and the amount excreted.
   (b) the area under the curve relating plasma concentration of a drug to time after administration.
   (c) the proportion of drug in a formulation that is found in the systemic circulation (plasma).
   (d) always idential with different formulations of the same drug.
   (e) a measure of the rate of absorption of a drug.

38 In general, drugs which are highly lipid soluble:
   (a) have low oil/water partition coefficients.
   (b) have high apparent volumes of distribution.
   (c) are readily absorbed from the gastrointestinal tract.
   (d) are readily excreted without being metabolized.
   (e) have very short elimination half-times.

36 (a) **True**   This is the definition of a single-compartment model.
   (b) **False** Although drug absorption often shows first order kinetics and a single exponential term will define the rise in plasma concentration, it does not necessarily follow that the drug is entering a single-compartment model. It is the number of exponential terms describing the drug *elimination* from the body that gives the number of compartments.
   (c) **False** This is not a prerequisite of a single-compartment model, only that the ratio of concentration in plasma and various tissues remains constant.
   (d) **False** See (c).
   (e) **False** A highly ionized drug *may* be restricted to the extracellular fluid but this does not necessarily mean that *all* drugs which are distributed in a single compartment are highly ionized.

37 (a) **False**
   (b) **False** This is amount of drug present in the plasma over a period of time.
   (c) **True**   This proportion of the dose administered is able to exert a pharmacological effect. Bioavailability is conventionally defined as the amount of drug found in plasma after administration by any other route, when compared with the amount of drug found in plasma when the same quantity of drug is given intravenously. The relative bioavailability (of different preparations given by the same or different routes) will compare the amount of drug found in plasma when different preparations of the drug are given by the same route or possibly by other routes.
   (d) **False** Different manufacturers' preparations of the same drug might have different bioavailabilities.
   (e) **False** But this may influence bioavailability, because, if absorption is slowed either from the gastrointestinal tract or from intramuscular injection sites, the drug may undergo degradation prior to absorption and less will be available for entry into the systemic circulation.

38 (a) **False** Drugs which are highly lipid soluble will tend to dissolve in oil rather than water.
   (b) **True**   Highly lipid-soluble drugs will penetrate most membranes easily and so enter most cells.
   (c) **True**   See (b).
   (d) **False** After filtration by the glomeruli, highly lipid-soluble drugs will tend to diffuse back into the body from the tubular fluid. Metabolism into more polar and less lipid-soluble substances will aid their excretion.
   (e) **False**

39 The renal clearance of a drug is much greater than the glomerular filtration
rate. This indicates that:
   (a) the renal clearance of the drug is less than that of creatinine.
   (b) the drug is actively secreted into the tubular fluid.
   (c) there is no renal tubular reabsorption.
   (d) the value of renal clearance is independent of the drug concentration
   in plasma.
   (e) the value of renal clearance of the drug may be higher than the renal
   clearance of para-aminohippuric acid (PAH).

40 The renal excretion of a drug will be reduced if:
   (a) the drug is a weak acid and the urinary pH is rendered acidic.
   (b) the drug is a weak base and the urinary pH is rendered alkaline.
   (c) the drug is amphetamine, and ammonium chloride has been administered.
   (d) the drug is aspirin, and sodium bicarbonate has been administered.
   (e) the drug is ethanol, and sodium bicarbonate has been administered.

41 In patients with reduced renal function (glomerular filtration rate < 50 ml/min)
the following drugs may cause the effects indicated:
   (a) aminoglycosides – ototoxicity.
   (b) digoxin – anorexia.
   (c) potassium-sparing diuretics – hyperkalaemia.
   (d) tetracycline – increased plasma urea.
   (e) tubocurarine – inadequate muscular relaxation.

39 (a) **False**   Clearance is defined as a volume from which a drug/substance is completely removed in unit time. Normal creatinine clearance is about 125 ml/min which means that creatinine is removed completely from 125 millilitres of blood or plasma each minute. If renal clearance of a drug is greater than the glomerular filtration rate it means that an additional process is operating to remove the drug from the blood or plasma; in other words active transport into the tubular fluid is occurring.

(b) **True**   See (a).

(c) **False**   You have no way of knowing whether this process is taking place or not; it would occur when clearance was maximal, i.e. equal to plasma flow through the kidney.

(d) **False**   As there is an active transport process involved it is possible to saturate this process.

(e) **False**   PAH is used to measure kidney plasma flow as its clearance is maximal; it is filtered and secreted but not reasorbed.

40 (a) **True**   A weak acid in an acidic urine will tend to be mainly undissociated and, as the undissociated moiety is more lipid soluble than the ionized chemical, it will tend to diffuse back into the circulation from the tubular fluid. Less will therefore be excreted.

(b) **True**   Similarly, a weak base in an alkaline urine will tend to be mainly undissociated.

(c) **False**   Amphetamine is a weak base and will be mainly ionized in urine rendered acidic by ammonium chloride. So, under these conditions, amphetamine will remain in the tubular fluid and will be excreted.

(d) **False**   Aspirin is a weak acid and will be mainly ionized in the presence of sodium bicarbonate, thus aiding excretion.

(e) **False**   The excretion of ethanol, which is neither acidic nor basic, is not influenced by changes in pH of the urine.

41 (a) **True**   Aminoglycosides such as neomycin and kanamycin can cause auditory impairment; streptomycin and gentamycin can produce vestibular toxicity. Aminoglycosides are excreted unchanged, mainly by glomerular filtration.

(b) **True**   Digoxin is eliminated 80–85 per cent unchanged by the kidney. Renal impairment is likely to raise the plasma concentration of digoxin to toxic levels, the earliest signs being anorexia and vomiting.

(c) **True**   Aldosterone causes Na^+ reabsorption and K^+ loss in the distal tubule. Spironolactone antagonizes this effect and is known as a potassium-sparing diuretic. In excessive dosage, or in renal impairment, this effect of spironolactone will be exaggerated and lead to hyperkalaemia.

(d) **True**   Tetracyclines (with few exceptions) are excreted unchanged in the urine. They have an anti-anabolic effect which raises blood urea and adds to the nitrogen load which requires excretion. In renal impairment the extra nitrogen load could cause further deterioration in renal function.

(e) **False**   Tubocurarine is partly excreted unchanged in the urine. With a severe degree of renal impairment prolonged paralysis will occur with large or repeated doses of the drug.

42 The following drugs are effective when swallowed:
    (a) glyceryl trinitrate.
    (b) diazepam.
    (c) (+) – tubocurarine.
    (d) insulin.
    (e) ampicillin.

43 The following statements about the distribution of drugs are true:
    (a) neostigmine readily crosses the blood-brain barrier.
    (b) lilpophilic drugs will cross the placental barrier.
    (c) tetracyclines are confined to the total body water.
    (d) drugs generally bind irreversibly to plasma proteins.
    (e) phenylbutazone can displace warfarin from plasma protein binding sites.

44 The following drugs pass readily across the blood-brain barrier:
    (a) promethazine.
    (b) aspirin.
    (c) naloxone.
    (d) L-DOPA.
    (e) dopamine.

42 (a) **False**   Glyceryl trinitrate is so extensively metabolized during its first passage through the liver that it does not reach the systemic circulation in sufficient amounts to cause detectable effects – an example of first pass metabolism. The drug is taken sublingually for buccal absoprtion, thereby reaching the general circulation before reaching the liver.

(b) **True**

(c) **False**   This is a quaternary ammonium compound which is highly ionized and relatively insoluble in lipid. Therefore the drug does not cross biological membranes readily and is ineffective when swallowed. Hence South American Indians can eat animals killed by arrows smeared with curare. The drug is injected intravenously to cause muscular relaxation during surgery.

(d) **False**   Insulin is a polypeptide which will be digested by enzymes in digestive juices. The drug is administered by injection.

(e) **True**   Unlike benzylpenicillin, it is not destroyed by gastric acid. (It is recommended that benzylpenicillin is taken orally on an empty stomach in order to reduce its destruction by gastric acid.)

43 (a) **False**   It is a quaternary ammonium compound extensively ionized in aqueous solution. The blood-brain barrier is virtually impermeable to such compounds.

(b) **True**

(c) **False**   Tetracyclines chelate calcium ions and so enter bone and teeth which are developing.

(d) **False**   Drugs generally bind reversibly with plasma proteins, particularly to albumin. An equilibrium is established between bound and non-bound drug. Only unbound drug is available for biological activity.

(e) **True**   This can be demonstrated *in vitro* and is one of the mechanisms offered as an explanation of the interaction of these drugs whereby the action of warfarin is enhanced.

44 (a) **True**   This is a histamine H_1-receptor antagonist and one of its actions is to cause drowsiness.

(b) **True**   It is effective in the treatment of headache! It also lowers elevated body temperature by acting in the hypothalamus.

(c) **True**   This is a competitive antagonist at opioid receptors, and is used to treat respiratory depression caused by morphine-like compounds. The respiratory-depressant effect of opiates is mediated by actions in the brain stem.

(d) **True**   L-DOPA is lipid soluble and crosses the blood-brain barrier by passive diffusion.

(e) **False**   Dopamine is not sufficiently lipid soluble to cross the blood-brain barrier. Peripherally it is taken up into many cells by uptake 2 where it is destroyed intracellularly by monoamine oxidase.

45 Drug metabolism can result in:
   (a) metabolites with greater water solubility than the parent compound.
   (b) glucuronidation.
   (c) metabolites with greater pharmacological activity than the parent compound.
   (d) metabolites with less pharmacological activity than the parent compound.
   (e) metabolites which are more readily excreted than the parent compound.

46 The therapeutic effects of the following drugs are made more active by metabolism:
   (a) suxamethonium.
   (b) paracetamol.
   (c) phenylephrine.
   (d) senna.
   (e) thiopentone.

47 In the following pairs of drug and enzyme, state whether the drug inhibits the enzyme:
   (a) physostigmine/plasma cholinesterase.
   (b) neostigmine/choline acetyltransferase.
   (c) botulinum toxin/acetylcholinesterase.
   (d) imipramine/monoamine oxidase.
   (e) reserpine/monoamine oxidase.

45 (a) **True** It is generally true that more water-soluble metabolites are more readily excreted by the kidney.

(b) **True** There may be two phases in drug metabolism. The first phase is a metabolic modification of the drug, for example oxidation, reduction or hydrolysis. The second phase is a synthetic reaction called conjugation which involves combination of the drug or metabolite with another molecule such as glucuronic acid or acetate.

(c) **True** Important examples are the conversion of codeine to morphine, L-DOPA to dopamine, and cortisone to hydrocortisone.

(d) **True** One example is the conversion by pseudocholinesterase of succinylcholine to succinylmonocholine, a metabolite with weaker action, before eventual complete hydrolysis.

(e) **True** See (a).

46 (a) **False** Suxamethonium (succinylcholine) is effectively two molecules of acetylcholine and is inactivated by plasma esterases; the acetylcholine formed is immediately inactivated by plasma esterases and acetylcholinesterases.

(b) **False** Paracetamol is metabolized to an epoxide which is normally conjugated to glutathione. Following toxic doses of paracetamol (10 g or more), the epoxide may bind to functional proteins in the liver when all the glutathione supply has been used up. This may lead to irreversible liver failure.

(c) **False** Phenylephrine is not converted into an active metabolite.

(d) **True** The major active constituents of the purgative senna are anthra-quinones, the glycosides of which are hydrolysed in the small intestine to liberate the quinones. These act on the large intestine which they reach via the blood supply after absorption in the small intestine or directly by passage through the gut lumen.

(e) **False** Thiopentone does not form active metabolites.

47 (a) **True** Physostigmine is a reversible competitive inhibitor of cholines-terase enzymes. It is used to enhance the effects of cholinergic nerve stimulation.

(b) **False** Neostigmine is another reversible competitive inhibitor of cholinesterase and is more stable and therefore longer lasting than physostigmine. Choline acetyltransferase is an enzyme which catalyzes synthesis of acetylcholine (acetylation of choline).

(c) **False** Botulinum toxin is produced by the anaerobic spore-forming bacterium clostridium botulinum, and prevents the release of acetylcholine by nerve impulses.

(d) **False** Imipramine is a tricyclic antidepressant and inhibits the neuronal uptake 1 process for noradrenaline thereby delaying its inactivation and potentiating its effects.

(e) **False** Reserpine prevents the active uptake of noradrenaline into storage vesicles in neurones. Reserpine chelates Mg^{2+}, which is required for the ATPase which energises the active transport process. Mg^{2+} also stabilizes the noradrenaline storage complex. Storage of other monoamines such as dopamine, 5-HT and adrenaline is also affected. Monoamine oxidase catalyses the oxidative deamination of a wide range of amines including catecholamines.

48 Adenylyl cyclase is:
- (a) a cyclic AMP inactivator.
- (b) a second messenger mediating the actions of some hormones.
- (c) regulated by G-proteins.
- (d) inhibited by theophylline at therapeutic concentrations.
- (e) activated via β-adrenoceptors.

49 Cyclic AMP:
- (a) is a neurotransmitter in the central nervous system.
- (b) activates kinases within cells.
- (c) is inactivated by uptake process.
- (d) synthesis can be caused by activation of β-adrenoceptors.
- (e) synthesis is inhibited by action of α_2-adrenoceptors.

48 (a) **False** It is an enzyme in the plasma membranes of many cells which catalyzes the conversion of ATP in the cytoplasm of cells to produce cyclic 3', 5'-AMP (c-AMP).

(b) **False** Cyclic AMP acts as a second messenger in the action of some hormones. A hormone (first messenger) occupies a receptor, adenylyl cyclase is activated, and C-AMP is formed. Cyclic AMP activates protein kinases which phosphorylate enzymes and other proteins. The activity of many such enzymes is regulated by their phosphorylation state; phosphorylation activates the enzymes, dephosphorylation inactivates them.

(c) **True** G-proteins (also known as regulatory proteins and N-proteins) act as a link between the primary messenger (hormone or neurotransmitter), the recognition site on the outer surface on the plasma membrane and the effector enzyme which generates the secondary messenger. They are called G-proteins because their activity is regulated by the binding of guanine nucleotides (GTP and GDP) which alter the affinity state of the G-protein for either the primary messenger binding site, or for the secondary messenger generating enzyme.

(d) **False** Theophylline, aminophylline, and caffeine are methylxanthines which at high concentrations can inhibit the enzymes which break down cyclic AMP. These enzymes are called phosphodiesterases. Until recently it was believed that the therapeutic action of these compounds was caused by the inhibition of phosphodiesterases and the subsequent accumulation of cyclic AMP. The concentration of methylxanthine necessary to inhibit phosphodiesterase is much higher than that which is achieved with any therapeutic dose of these compounds. Methylxanthines are competitive inhibitors at P2 purinergic receptors and it is likely that this accounts for their therapeutic activity as bronchodilators, diuretics, and mild central nervous stimulants.

(e) **True** Some of the metabolic effects of adrenaline and noradrenaline are produced by activating adenylyl cyclase via β-adrenoceptors.

49 (a) **False** It is a secondary messenger inside cells.

(b) **True** Kinases are enzymes which phosphorylate either other enzymes or other proteins. Phosphorylation is a common mechanism for activation of enzymes and proteins.

(c) **False** It is inactivated by phosphodiesterases. Inhibitors of phosphodiesterases can increase the concentration of cyclic AMP and prolong its duration of action within cells. At therapeutic doses methylxanthines, for example caffeine and aminophylline, do not inhibit phosphodiesterases.

(d) **True** Activation of β-adrenoceptors (by agonists such as adrenaline, noradrenaline, isoprenaline or salbutamol) leads to activation of the enzyme adenylyl cyclase which catalyses the conversion of ATP into cyclic AMP. The binding site for agonists in β-adrenoceptors is linked to adenylyl cyclase by a stimulatory G protein (Gs).

(e) **True** α_2-adrenoceptors are linked to adenylyl cyclase by an inhibitory G protein (Gi). Activation of α_2-adrenoceptors by noradrenaline, clonidine, or α-methylnoradrenaline, leads to reduced synthesis of cyclic AMP.

50 The enzyme phospholipase C:
  (a) cleaves arachidonic acid from membrane triglyceride.
  (b) is regulated by G proteins.
  (c) activation can lead to liberation of intracellular calcium.
  (d) is inhibited by macrocortin.
  (e) phosphorylates G proteins

51 G proteins (also called regulatory proteins):
  (a) can regulate the opening state of ion channels.
  (b) are involved in the transduction of hormonal signals.
  (c) are unaffected by the actions of bacterial toxins.
  (d) are regulated in part by availability of ATP.
  (e) regulate the opening of nicotinic acetylcholine-receptor-operated channels.

50 (a) **False**   It liberates inositol trisphosphate from membrane triglyceride. The enzyme phospholipase A_2 liberates arachidonic acid from membrane trigylcerides.

(b) **True**   Phospholipase C is an enzyme which is linked to binding sites for some neurotransmitters and hormones by stimulatory G proteins (Gs).

(c) **True**   Inositol trisphosphate, liberated by the action of phospholipase C, is an intracellular secondary messenger which acts at recognition sites in the endoplasmic reticulum, this regulates release of calcium from the endoplasmic reticulum. Changes in intracellular calcium lead to increased activity of enzymes and other proteins.

(d) **False**   Macrocortin is a protein which inhibits phospholipase A_2 but not phospholipase C.

51 (a) **True**   In addition to regulating the activity of enzymes adenylyl cyclase and phospholipase C, some G proteins work within the plasma membrane of cells to regulate opening of ion channels in the membrane.

(b) **True**   G proteins link the binding site for primary messengers, which is found on the outside of cells, to the effector mechanisms either in the cell membrane (see option (a) above), or to effector enzymes on the cytoplasmic site of the cell membrane. Primary messengers include hormones and neurotransmitters.

(c) **False**   Pertussis (whooping cough) toxin irreversibly inhibits some classes of inhibitory G proteins. By contrast cholera toxin irreversibly activates some classes of stimulatory G proteins. These toxins are used as research tools and the irreversible nature of their action explains the potentially serious toxic effects when infection occurs with agents secreting these toxins.

(d) **False**   G proteins are so called because their activity is regulated by the high-energy compound guanine triphosphate and guanine diphosphate. Binding of an agonist to the recognition site associated with the G protein increases the affinity of the G protein for GTP. When GTP binds to the G protein, the G protein dissociates and can interact with either ion channels or enzymes which regulate the synthesis of secondary messengers.

(e) **False**   Nicotinic receptors for acetylcholine are found on the proteins which form the transmembrane cation channel whose state of opening is regulated by acetycholine. This is a very fast responding transduction mechanism, and G proteins are not associated with it. Transduction mechanisms which involve G proteins are slower than those involving ligand-regulated ion channels.

52 The activity of liver microsomal enzymes:
   (a) is important in the metabolism of barbiturates.
   (b) can be inhibited by monoamine oxidase inhibitors.
   (c) can be induced by some anticonvulsant drugs.
   (d) can alter the activity of coumarin anticoagulants.
   (e) is induced by morphine.

53 The following statements about the excretion of drugs are correct:
   (a) ampicillin is found in bile.
   (b) halothane is excreted by the lungs.
   (c) glucuronidated metabolites may be excreted in the bile.
   (d) ethanol can be found in milk.
   (e) probenicid can reduce the excretion of penicillin in urine.

52 (a) **True**   The liver is a major site of drug metabolism, although metabolism can occur in other tissues. The microsomal enzymes are a heterogeneous collection of enzymes which can be separated by high speed centrifugation.

(b) **True**   Whereas MAO is found on mitochondria, amine oxidases are also found among the microsomal enzymes. Further, MAO inhibitors are not specific for just MAO, as they can inhibit other enzymes.

(c) **True**   Enzyme induction is a process whereby a stimulus – in this case an anticonvulsant drug, e.g. phenytoin or phenobarbitone – initiates extra synthesis of enzymes.

(d) **True**   Coumarin anticoagulants are inactivated by metabolism by liver microsomal enzymes. If enzyme activity is decreased, then metabolism will be slowed and anticoagulant activity will increase. The converse is true if microsomal enzymes are induced.

(e) **True**   However, whilst some induction of enzymes which metabolize morphine does occur, most of the tolerance developed cannot be explained in this way, and is probably due to adaptation of receptors in the nervous system to the action of the drug.

53 (a) **True**   It is actively secreted into bile, which is useful in some biliary tract infections. Drugs excreted into bile pass into the intestine from which reabsorption can occur – enterohepatic circulation.

(b) **True**   Some halothane (about 15 per cent) is also metabolized by the liver. Chloride and bromide ions are removed from halothane and the urine contains organic fluorine-containing compounds.

(c) **True**   An active transport system exists in the liver for biliary excretion of endogenous glucuronides, and many glucuronides are excreted using this mechanism.

(d) **True**

(e) **True**   Renal excretion of penicillin is largely a tubular-secretion mechanism. Probenicid competes with penicillin for the carrier and so prolongs the plasma half-time and duration of action of penicillins.

54 The figure below shows log dose – response curves for drugs R and S and R in the presence of T. all of which act on the same receptors. On the basis of the date provided, indicate whether or not the following statements are true.
  (a) R and S have the same efficacy.
  (b) S is a full agonist.
  (c) At 50 per cent maximum response, R is more potent than S.
  (d) S is a competitive antagonist of R.
  (e) T is a competitive antagonist of R.

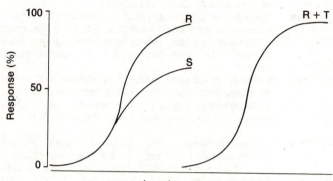

Log dose of agonist

55 Which of the following statements about receptor-operated (ligand-operated) ion channels is/are true:
  (a) nicotinic receptors are coupled to sodium ion channels.
  (b) muscarinic receptors are coupled to sodium ion channels.
  (c) α_1-adrenoceptors in the gut are directly coupled to a calcium ion channel.
  (d) NMDA (N-methyl-D-aspartic acid) receptors are directly linked to a cation channel.
  (e) activation of GABA A receptors closes chloride ion channels.

54 (a) **False**   Efficacy is defined as the ability to produce a given response. S can only produce about 50 per cent of the maximum achievable response, thus it has a lower efficacy than R.

(b) **False**   R is a full agonist – it can produce a 100 per cent response. S is a partial agonist.

(c) **True**   Potency is a measure of the quantity of drug needed to produce a defined response. The log dose of R to produce a 50 per cent maximal response is less than the log dose of S to produce the same effect.

(d) **False**   We know nothing about the possible antagonist action of S, as we have no details of the response which occurs when the two drugs are present at the same time.

(e) **True**   In the presence of T, the dose-response curve to R has (i) been displaced to the right, (ii) remained parallel to the dose-response curve to R alone, (iii) achieved the same maximum response. With these three conditions satisfied, it is concluded that T is a competitive antagonist of R.

55 (a) **True**   Receptor-regulated ion channels incorporate a ligand binding site which, when occupied by an appropriate messenger molecule, induces a conformational change in the channel protein which opens an ion-specific channel. Nicotinic acetyl-choline receptors on skeletal muscle in ganglia, and in the central nervous system, regulate the opening of a cation channel which is permeable to sodium and potassium. Influx of sodium ions leads to depolarisation of the membrane and initiates a chain of events leading to excitatory responses such as muscular contraction or generation of action potentials.

(b) **False**   All muscarinic receptors are linked to their effector mechanism by a G protein. This contrasts with the fast receptor-operated ion channels (see (a) above and (e) below) in which the neurotrans-mitter recognition site is an integral part of the ion channel. Muscarinic receptors in the heart, some smooth muscles, and in the central nervous system are linked to potassium ion channels. This linkage is effected by a G protein which is activated within the plasma membrane when the muscarinic recognition site is occupied by an appropriate agonist; in these circumstances the G protein facilitates opening of potassium ion channels. Opening of K^+ channels leads to hyperpolarisation of the cell membrane. This inhibitory effect leads to decreased excitability of the cell membrane.

(c) **False**   Receptor-operated calcium ion channels for conventional neurotransmitters have not been described. All α-adrenoceptors are members of the G protein-regulated super family of receptors.

(d) **True**   NMDA receptors are receptors for the excitatory amino acids, glutamic acid and aspartic acid, in the central nervous system. The recognition site forms part of the ion channel and occupation of the recognition site by excitatory amino acids leads to opening of the cation channel which allows entry of sodium ions and calcium ions into the cell.

(e) **False**   GABA A receptors are an integral part of a chloride ion channel which opens when the GABA A recognition site is occupied by an agonist molecule. This leads to entry of chloride ions into the cell and causes hyperpolarisation.

56 Competitive antagonists:
   (a) produce their effects by binding to different types of receptors than do their respective agonists.
   (b) have lower dissociation rate constants than respective agonists.
   (c) alter the slope of the log dose-response curve of an agonist.
   (d) cause the log dose-response curve to be shifted to the left.
   (e) must block all receptors to cause antagonism.

57 The following drug combinations demonstrate physiological antagonism:
   (a) isoprenaline and histamine on bronchioles.
   (b) salbutamol and propranolol on bronchioles.
   (c) acetylcholine and adrenaline on the heart.
   (d) phenylephrine and acetylcholine on the pupil.
   (e) physostigmine and pilocarpine on the ciliary muscle.

56 (a) **False** Competitive antagonists and their respective agonists compete for the same receptors.

  (b) **True** Competitive antagonists dissociate from receptors slowly and thus fewer receptors are available for interaction with the agonist.

  (c) **False** In the presence of a competitive antagonist, a log dose-response curve to the agonist can be obtained by increasing all the doses of the agonist by the same multiple. The slope is unchanged, the same maximum response to the agonist. can be obtained, and the log dose-response curve in the presence of the competitive antagonist is parallel to that obtained in the absence of the antagonist.

  (d) **False** Such a movement would indicate potentiation. In fact, the log dose-response curve will move to the right and will be parallel to the original curve.

  (e) **False** It is only necessary for a fraction of receptors to be blocked in order to demonstrate competitive antagonism. If the concentration of agonist is increased, the rate of interaction of agonist with the reduced number of free receptors will be such that the original response can be obtained.

57 (a) **True** Physiological antagonism operates when two agonists act on a single tissue to produce opposite physiological effects. Histamine acting at H_1-receptors causes bronchoconstriction; isoprenaline acting on β-adrenoceptors causes bronchodilatation.

  (b) **False** Competitive antagonism occurs when a competitive inhibitor at a single receptor blocks access at that receptor to an agonist. Propranolol is a competitive antagonist (of salbutamol) at β-adrenoceptors in the bronchi.

  (c) **True** Acetylcholine acts at muscarinic receptors and adrenaline acts at β-adrenoceptors to cause slowing and speeding of the heart respectively; this is a form of physiological antagonism.

  (d) **True** Phenylephrine and acetylcholine act at α_1 and muscarinic receptors to have antagonistic actions on the pupil.

  (e) **False** Physostigmine is a reversible competitive inhibitor of acetylcholinesterase and so increases the amount of acetylcholine present in the synaptic cleft. Pilocarpine is a muscarinic receptor agonist. Effects of the two drugs will be additive at least, and there will be no antagonism.

58 In the following pairs of drugs, indicate whether the first substance increases the effects of the second *in vivo*:
   (a) spironolactone/aldosterone.
   (b) tranyclypromine/amphetamine.
   (c) promethazine/ethanol.
   (d) phenobarbitone/warfarin.
   (e) tranylcypromine/pethidine.

59 In the following pairs of drugs, indicate whether the first substance increases the action of the second in vivo:
   (a) hexamethonium/suxamethonium.
   (b) neostigmine/(+)-tubocurarine.
   (c) imipramine/noradrenaline.
   (d) physostigmine/atropine.
   (e) physostigmine/acetylcholine.

58 (a) **False**   Spironolactone is a competitive antagonist of aldosterone.

(b) **True**   Tranylcypromine is a MAO inhibitor which increases the concentration of monoamine within nerves. Amphetamine displaces monoamines from nerves and if higher than normal concentrations of monoamines exist in the nerves (as occurs following treatment with tranylcypromine), then the effects of amphetamine will be enhanced.

(c) **True**   Promethazine and ethanol are CNS depressants which means that they can cause respiratory depression. The respiratory depressant effects of promethazine and ethanol are additive and can prove fatal.

(d) **False**   Phenobarbitone is a powerful inducer of microsomal enzymes. Warfarin is inactivated by microsomal enzymes, so that the rate of metabolism of warfarin may be speeded up if there is increased microsomal enzyme activity following exposure to phenobarbitone.

(e) **True**   Pethidine is metabolized by microsomal enzymes, and this in part terminates its action in the body. In addition to inhibiting monoamine oxidase, tranylcypromine inhibits mcrosomal enzymes and so decreases metabolism of pethidine.

59 (a) **False**   Hexamethonium is a competitive antagonist at nicotinic receptors in autonomic ganglia. Suxamethonium is an open channel blocker at nicotinic receptors at the neuromuscular junction. The drugs have some selectivity for the nicotinic receptor subtypes upon which they act and no interactions occur between them.

(b) **False**   Neostigmine is a competitive inhibitor of the enzyme acetylcholinesterase in the synaptic cleft where it prevents the breakdown of acetylcholine. Tubocurarine is a competitive antagonist at nicotinic receptors in skeletal muscle. Neostigmine increases the concentration of acetylcholine at this site which would tend to reverse the effectiveness of (+)-tubocurarine by displacing it from the nicotinic receptors.

(c) **True**   Imipramine is an inhibitor of uptake 1 into sympathetic nerve terminals. Noradrenaline in the synaptic cleft is inactivated by neuronal uptake 1. In the presence of imipramine, the concentration of noradrenaline and its duration of stay in the synaptic cleft will be increased. Therefore imipramine enhances the action of noradrenaline.

(d) **False**   Atropine is a muscarinic receptor blocker. Physostigmine is an inhibitor of acetylcholinesterase. Physostigmine will increase the concentration of acetylcholine in the synaptic cleft which will tend to displace atropine from muscarinic receptors, thus leading to a decreased effect of atropine.

(e) **True**   As described above, physostigmine is an anticholinesterase; it will enhance the actions of acetylcholine because it prevents its breakdown by the enzyme acetylcholinesterase.

60 Mast cells:
   (a) contain histamine.
   (b) synthesize antigens.
   (c) are present in intestinal vascular tisseue.
   (d) can release leucotrienes.
   (e) are stabilized by herparin.

61 The following are used to treat bronchial asthma:
   (a) β_2-adrenoceptor agonists.
   (b) histamine H_1-receptor blockers.
   (c) inhibitors of prostaglandin synthesis.
   (d) prostaglandin receptor blockers.
   (e) muscarinic receptor blockers.

62 Disodium cromoglycate (DSCG):
   (a) is well absorbed from the gastrointestinal tract.
   (b) stabilizes mast cells and prevents their degranulation.
   (c) is inhaled as a powder for prophylaxis of bronchial asthma.
   (d) can cause bronchoconstriction during administration.
   (e) is used in the treatment of allergic rhinitis.

60 (a) **True**   Mast cells release histamine on antigen challenge. Mast cells have membrane receptors to which IgE antibodies bind. When a specific antigen reaches a mast cell and binds to the receptor, bound IgE antibody, histamine, serotonin, prostaglandins and leucotrienes are released.

(b) **False**

(c) **True**   Mast cells are found in connective tissue around blood vessels and lymphatics, particularly in the lungs, liver and intestines.

(d) **True**   On antigen challenge, mast cells can release a variety of substances including histamine, serotonin, prostaglandins and leucotrienes (including SRS-A).

(e) **False**   Mast cells contain heparin, an anticoagulant which prevents clot formation after injury. Cromoglycate, an antiallergic drug prevents the release of mediators from mast cells, and is said to stabilize mast cells.

61 (a) **True**   β-adrenoceptor agonists cause bronchodilatation. Salbutamol is a selective agonist at these receptors and is preferable to isoprenaline.

(b) **False**   In allergic asthma, a variety of pharmacologically active substances including histamine, slow-reacting substance of anaphylaxis (SRS-A) and prostaglandins are released from mast cells. Antihistamines are ineffective presumably because histamine is only one of several substances causing broncho-constriction, and SRS-A is considered to be the main agent causing bronchoconstriction in asthmatics. A more effective remedy is a β-adrenoceptor agonist acting as a physiological antagonist against all the bronchoconstrictor agents.

(c) **False**   See (b).

(d) **False**   See (b).

(e) **True**   However, such drugs have side-effects by actions on other muscarinic receptors; ipratropium may be useful in patients with airway obstruction caused by chronic bronchitis.

62 (a) **False**

(b) **True**   The antigen-induced release of substances such as SRS-A and histamine from human mast cells is reduced by DSCG. It is used prophylactically.

(c) **True**   Persons taking DSCG must learn to inhale the powder from a specially designed dispenser. DSCG is also available as an aerosol inhalation.

(d) **True**   This is usually transient and is caused by the mechanical irritation of inhaling a powder.

(e) **True**

63 Steroids with glucocorticoid activity:
  (a) include beclomethasone.
  (b) have a rapid onset of action when used in status asthmaticus.
  (c) do not have anti-inflammatory activity.
  (d) can be taken orally.
  (e) when given to treat bronchial asthma, do not depress pituitary function.

64 The following may induce bronchospasm:
  (a) noradrenaline.
  (b) morphine.
  (c) acetylcholine.
  (d) slow-reacting substance of anaphylaxis (SRS-A).
  (e) ephedrine.

65 The following statements about the anti-inflammatory analgesics indicated are true:
  (a) aspirin is valuable in the treatment of gastrointestinal pain.
  (b) paracetamol is a potent anti-inflammatory agent.
  (c) salicylates are effective in the treatment of rheumatoid arthritis.
  (d) indomethacin can displace warfarin from plasma proteins.
  (e) aspirin has antipyretic activity.

66 Naproxen:
  (a) is a propionic acid derivative:
  (b) has a shorter plasma half-life than aspirin.
  (c) is preferred to aspirin for treatment of acute gout.
  (d) can cause aplastic anaemia.
  (e) can cause gastric bleeding.

63 (a) **True**   This is a fluorinated steroid used in asthma in the form of an aerosol. A metered dose is delivered to the lungs and the possibility of systemic effects is reduced – but, see (e).

  (b) **False**   They must be used prophylactically. They have several effects including reduction of the release of mediators, thus they will not stop status asthmaticus once it is established.

  (c) **False**   Prednisolone and dexamethasone are used for their anti-inflammatory actions.

  (d) **True**   They can also be injected, applied topically, and some can be inhaled.

  (e) **False**   Suppression of ACTH secretion by the pituitary is a major adverse effect of glucocorticoid therapy, causing inadequate adrenal steroid response to stress with life-threatening consequences.

64 (a) **False**   Noradrenaline is the endogenous neurotransmitter acting at β_2-adrenoceptors in the bronchioles causing dilatation.

  (b) **True**   It causes bronchoconstriction by releasing histamine.

  (c) **True**

  (d) **True**   This is believed to be one of the major mediators of anaphylactic bronchospasm.

  (e) **False**   This sympathomimetic amine causes bronchodilatation mainly by an indirect action.

65 (a) **False**   Aspirin can cause or exacerbate gastrointestinal pains. It causes gastric ulceration and is ineffective in reducing gut pain.

  (b) **False**   In contrast to aspirin, paracetamol has no anti-inflammatory action.

  (c) **True**   They decrease both pain and inflammation.

  (d) **True**   This can lead to increased anticoagulant effect (warfarin).

  (e) **True**

66 (a) **True**

  (b) **False**   When used to treat inflammation aspirin needs to be taken about every 4 hours; by contrast naproxen can be taken twice daily only.

  (c) **True**   Naproxen causes fewer adverse effects than aspirin; when high doses are given frequently, as in acute gout, this is a special advantage.

  (d) **False**   Phenylbutazone occasionally causes this adverse effect.

  (e) **True**   This side effect occurs occasionally.

67 Prostaglandins:
   (a) may be involved in the mediation of inflammation.
   (b) are believed to mediate the febrile response.
   (c) can induce labour.
   (d) synthesis is inhibited by aspirin.
   (e) can cause both bronchoconstriction and bronchodilatation.

68 Thromboxane A_2:
   (a) is a prostaglandin.
   (b) synthesis is inhibited by aspirin.
   (c) has a half-life of 5 minutes.
   (d) causes platelet aggregation.
   (e) causes vasodilatation.

69 Plasma cholesterol can be reduced by:
   (a) binding bile acids in the gut with an anion-exchange resin.
   (b) nicotinic acid.
   (c) clofibrate.
   (d) tyramine.
   (e) polystyrene sulphonate resin.

67 (a) **True**   Prostaglandins (and other pharmacologically active substances) are released in inflammatory reactions and mediate some aspects of the inflammatory response.

(b) **True**   Injection of prostaglandin E_1 into the cerebral ventricles produces an increase in body temperature. In endotoxin-induced fever, the prostaglandin concentration in cerebrospinal fluid rises and this rise is prevented by drugs inhibiting prostaglandin synthesis.

(c) **True**   Prostaglandin E_2 can be used for this purpose.

(d) **True**   Aspirin and some other anti-inflammatory drugs prevent the synthesis of prostaglandins from arachidonic acid by inhibiting the cyclo-oxygenase enzyme.

(e) **True**   In general, prostaglandins of the F series contract and those of the E series relax bronchial muscle. Asthmatics are particularly sensitive to the bronchoconstrictor effect of prostaglandin $F_{2\alpha}$.

68 (a) **False**   Thromboxane A_2 is a metabolite of cyclic endoperoxides; the prostaglandin cyclopentane ring is replaced by a six membered oxygen containing ring.

(b) **True**   Aspirin inhibits the cyclo-oxygenase enzyme system which converts arachidonic acid to cyclic endoperoxides which are then converted to prostaglandins and thromboxane.

(c) **False**   Thromboxane A_2 has a half-life of about 30 seconds and is converted to the biologically inactive thromboxane B_2.

(d) **True**   Thromboxane A_2 is one of the most potent platelet aggregators known.

(e) **False**   Thromboxane A_2 causes vasoconstriction.

69 (a) **True**   Cholestryamine is an anion-exchange resin that binds bile acids which are formed from cholesterol in the liver and secreted into the intestine. The bile acids are excreted in the faeces thus depleting the bile acid pool. This depletion stimulates the conversion of cholesterol to bile acid and the result is that the concentration of plasma low-density lipoprotein cholesterol falls by 20 to 25 per cent.

(b) **True**   Nicotinic acid lowers plasma triglyceride and cholesterol concentrations. It is used to treat hyperlipidaemia and probably acts as anti lipolytic agent in adipose tissue reducing the supply of non-esterified free fatty acids and hence the substrate for hepatic lipoprotein synthesis.

(c) **True**   Clofibrate inhibits hepatic lipid synthesis. Plasma cholesterol and triglyceride decline, see (a).

(d) **False**   Cholestyramine is used to reduce plasma cholesterol, see (a). Tyramine is a sympathomimetic amine.

(e) **False**   Polystyrene sulphonate resin is a cation-exchange resin used in hyperkalaemia to prevent absorption of ingested potassium from the gut.

70 Cardiac glycosides:
   (a) increase vagal effects on the heart.
   (b) increase excitability of ventricular muscle.
   (c) increase conduction in the bundle of His.
   (d) can induce atrial fibrillation.
   (e) have a high therapeutic ratio.

71 Cardiac glycosides:
   (a) improve the efficiency of the heart.
   (b) are used in the treatment of congestive heart failure.
   (c) can be given orally or intravenously.
   (d) can cause a decrease in ventricular rate.
   (e) are used to treat ventricular dysrhythmias.

72 Indicate whether the following can modify the action of digoxin.
   (a) sympathomimetic amines.
   (b) chlorothiazide.
   (c) poor kidney function.
   (d) quinidine.
   (e) increased plasma levels of Ca^{2+}.

70 (a) **True**   These vagal effects on the heart appear to involve at least three mechanisms:
  (i) slowing of pacemaker cells in the sinoatrial node,
  (ii) slowing of the rate of conduction of impulses between atria and ventricles (in the bundle of His).
  (iii) decrease in atrial refractory period which therefore speeds repolarization of atrial cells, and leads to weaker contractions of the atria. It is not clear whether cardiac glycosides alter the sensitivity of muscarinic receptors in the heart, or whether the actions are mediated centrally using the baroreceptor pathways.

  (b) **True**   This is an undesirable property of these compounds and can cause ventricular dysrhythmias.

  (c) **False** Conductions in the bundle of His are slowed by a direct action, and also indirectly via the enhanced vagal activity. See (a).

  (d) **True**   This may be a sign of toxicity.

  (e) **False**

71 (a) **True**   The amount of work done by the heart for unit consumption of oxygen is increased.

  (b) **True**

  (c) **True**   Digoxin oral or intravenously; ouabain intravenous only.

  (d) **True**   In heart failure, there is usually an elevated ventricular heart rate, and this is reduced by cardiac glycosides partly by indirect actions through vagal mechanisms and partly by a reduction in the compensatory tachycardia as a result of improvement in cardiac function. See (a).

  (e) **False** Whereas atrial dysrhythmias can be treated with cardiac glycosides, ventricular dysrhythmias occur at toxic levels as a result of increased cardiac excitability and automaticity.

72 (a) **True**   Sympathomimetic amines can increase cardiac excitability and automaticity which can lead to dysrhythmias.

  (b) **True**   Chlorothiazide is a diuretic which causes K^+ loss. The toxicity of cardiac glycosides (especially their dysrhythmic effects) is increased in hypokalaemia.

  (c) **True**   As digoxin is largely removed from the body by excretion through the kidney, in kidney failure there may be a slowing of its excretion, which can lead to toxicity. Digitoxin is inactivated mainly by the liver and so is safer than digoxin in renal failure, though it should be remembered that one of the metabolites of digitoxin is digoxin.

  (d) **True**   Quinidine displaces digoxin from plasma protein-binding sites, and digoxin actions are potentiated.

  (e) **True**   The actions of cardiac glycosides can be mimicked by Ca^{2+}, thus when combined, potentiation occurs. This is important if calcium must be given intravenously to digitalized patients.

73 The following drugs relieve angina. They do so for the reasons stated.
   (a) glyceryl trinitrate – by reducing left ventricular work.
   (b) glyceryl trinitrate – by causing dilatation of extra-cardiac blood vessels.
   (c) propranolol – by decreasing sympathetic tone of the heart.
   (d) amyl nitrite – by causing dilatation of the coronary arteries.
   (e) amyl nitrite – by inhibiting the uptake of calcium by myocardial cells.

74 Glyceryl trinitrate:
   (a) is the treatment of choice in congestive heart failure.
   (b) has to be converted to a nitrite before it is effective.
   (c) has a duration of action of several hours following buccal absorption.
   (d) can cause a fall in blood pressure.
   (e) can increase exercise tolerance if taken immediately before exercise.

75 Isosorbide dinitrate:
   (a) is effective sublingually.
   (b) is effective when swallowed.
   (c) produces active metabolites.
   (d) is useful for prophylaxis in angina.
   (e) has a shorter duration of action than glyceryl trinitrate.

76 The following drugs control cardiac dysrhythmias by the mechanisms
   indicated:
   (a) lignocaine decreases the rate of rapid depolarization of cardiac cells.
   (b) propranolol has local anesthetic activity.
   (c) practolol has β-adrenoceptor blocking properties.
   (d) phenytoin blocks the calcium current component of depolarization of
       cardiac tissue.
   (e) amiodarone prolongs the refractory period of the cardiac action potential.

73 (a) **True**   Nitrates and nitrites cause dilatation of veins and venules. This leads to peripheral pooling of blood and decreased venous return to the heart. The workload of the heart is reduced.

(b) **True**   See (a).

(c) **True**   An increase in sympathetic tone in response to exercise leads to an increase in the oxygen requirement of the heart. In angina, this leads to ischaemic pain. Propranolol is a β-adrenoceptor blocker and decreases cardiac response to sympathetic stimulation.

(d) **False**   Whereas coronary vasodilatation to nitrates can be demonstrated in isolated heart preparations and in experimental animals, the explanation for the relief obtained in angina is primarily due to a decrease in cardiac work secondary to the fall in systemic blood pressure. See (a).

(e) **False**   Drugs exerting such activity include verapamil and prenylamine, and they are used as antidysrhythmics.

74 (a) **False**   The conventional treatment is the use of cardiac glycosides. There has been some evaluation of the use of nitrates in acute refractory congestive failure but certainly they are not as reliably effective as cardiac glycosides for chronic treatment of congestive heart failure.

(b) **False**

(c) **False**   Following buccal absorption, glyceryl trinitrate is usually effective within 2 minutes in alleviating an anginal attack, and is effective for about 30 minutes.

(d) **True**   Dizziness and fainting are commonly reported side effects. Headache also occurs and may be due to stretching of meningeal structures by the increased pulsations resulting from cerebral vasodilatation.

(e) **True**   Anginal pain may be prevented if the drug is used prophylactically before exercise or stress.

75 (a) **True**

(b) **True**

(c) **True**   The most important of the active metabolites is isosorbide mononitrate.

(d) **True**

(e) **False**   Isosorbide dinitrate has a slower onset of action than glyceryl trinitrate but its action may persist for several hours. A duration of action of up to 12 hours is claimed for sustained-release preparations.

76 (a) **True**   It also increases the threshold at which pacemaker cells discharge.

(b) **False**   It is the β-adrenoceptor blocking action of propranolol which is the major contribution to its antidysrhythmic action.

(c) **True**   This now remains the major use of this drug.

(d) **False**   Phenytoin has local anaesthetic activity which is responsible for its antidysrhythmic action. Verapamil and prenylamine block calcium channels and reduce the entry of calcium.

(e) **True**

77 Lignocaine:
  (a) is given orally when it is used to control cardiac dysrhythmias.
  (b) has vasoconstrictor properties.
  (c) does not penetrate the blood-brain barrier.
  (d) is an effective local anaesthetic when applied to mucous membranes.
  (e) is inactivated by plasma cholinesterases.

78 Coumarin anticoagulants:
  (a) are effective within minutes of administration.
  (b) can be displaced from plasma protein-binding sites by aspirin..
  (c) are used for their actions *in vitro*.
  (d) include ancrod.
  (e) may be more rapidly metabolized in patients taking barbiturates.

79 Heparin is an anticoagulant which:
  (a) is effective when swallowed.
  (b) produced its anticoagulant effect primarily by reducing platelet adhesive-
     ness.
  (c) is effective *in vitro*.
  (d) is antagonized by vitamin K.
  (e) is potentiated by protamine.

77 (a) **False**   It is administered intravenously to control ventricular dysrhythmias. This drug undergoes hepatic first pass metabolism and would have to be given too frequently by the oral route to maintain a constant blood concentration.

  (b) **False**   Lignocaine is combined with the vasoconstrictor adrenaline to provide an adequate duration of local anaesthesia.

  (c) **False**   Stimulation, followed by depression, of the CNS is a hazard of its use intravenously.

  (d) **True**   The unionized form is lipid soluble and penetrates cell membranes.

  (e) **False**   Procaine is inactivated in this way, lignocaine is metabolized in the liver.

78 (a) **False**   Dicoumarol and warfarin block the formation of clotting factors in the liver; thus about 24 hours elapse before an anticoagulant effect is evident.

  (b) **True**   This can lead to an increase in free anticoagulant in the plasma, and result in bleeding, especially in the gut and kidneys.

  (c) **False**   See (a).

  (d) **False**   Ancrod is used as an alternative to heparin. It is an enzyme which reduces plasma fibrinogen by cleavage of fibrin.

  (e) **True**   Coumarins are inactivated by liver microsomal enzymes, which can be induced by barbiturates.

79 (a) **False**   It is an acidic mucopolysaccharide which is precipitated by gastric acid. Being of large molecular weight, it does not cross membranes easily and, presumably the small amount that might be absorbed would be metabolized in the liver. It is injected intravenously.

  (b) **False**   In large doses, heparin does inhibit platelet aggregation caused by thrombin, but the main action of heparin is as described in (c).

  (c) **True**   Heparin increases the activity of antithrombin III, a substance present in plasma which is an inhibitor of clotting factors, e.g. factor X and thrombin.

  (d) **False**   Warfarin and dicoumarol interfere with the formation of various clotting factors from vitamin K. Hence vitamin K will antagonize the anticoagulant effect of these two drugs but not heparin, which has a different mode of action – see (c).

  (e) **False**   Protamine, a strongly basic protein obtained from fish sperm, combines with heparin, which is strongly acidic, to form a stable complex devoid of anticoagulant action.

80 The following drugs cause diuresis by the mechanisms indicated:
    (a) ethanol – by preventing the reabsorption of Na^+ from renal tubular fluid.
    (b) digitalis – by inhibiting the release of antidiuretic hormone.
    (c) dopamine – by increasing renal blood flow.
    (d) frusemide – by inhibiting carbonic anhydrase.
    (e) chlorothiazide – by inhibiting active sodium transport in the ascending loop of Henle.

81 The following statements about diuretics are correct:
    (a) antidiuretic hormone (ADH) is used to treat diabetes insipidus.
    (b) chlorothiazide is used in the treatment of gout.
    (c) frusemide has greater efficacy than chlorothiazide.
    (d) thiazide diuretics may be used safely by persons with diabetes mellitus.
    (e) low doses of intravenous dopamine can cause a diuresis.

80 (a) **False** Ethanol blocks the secretion of antidiuretic hormone.

   (b) **False** Diuresis following treatment with digitalis is due to increased cardiac output, which results in improved perfusion of the kidneys.

   (c) **True** See 81 (e).

   (d) **False** Frusemide is a 'loop diuretic' see 81(c). Acetazolamide is a carbonic anhydrase inhibitor with weak diuretic activity. Inhibition of carbonic anhydrase reduces the supply of H^+ in the distal tubule where it is exchanged for reabsorbed Na^+. The result is an increased Na^+ excretion with accompanying water.

   (e) **True** The precise location of the main action of this drug is in the cortical segment of the ascending loop of Henle. An increased excretion of Na^+, accompanied by Cl^-, and HCO_3^- and water results. As a consequence of the increased load of Na^+ in the distal tubule, a loss of K^+ occurs.

81 (a) **True** Diabetes insipidus, in which the urine is dilute and tasteless, results from a lack of ADH. The permeability of the collecting tubules in the kidney to water is increased by ADH.

   (b) **False** Diuretics which ·block active transport of ions out of the kidney tubules, may also block the secretion of uric acid into the kidney tubules. As deposition of uric is the cause of gout, anything which inhibits its excretion can bring about this condition.

   (c) **True** Frusemide inhibits active transport of Cl^- over the entire length of the ascending loop of Henle (loop diuretic). The dose-response curve is steep, unlike the thiazides, and up to 30 per cent of the total sodium content of the glomerular filtrate does not get reabsorbed. Loop diuretics have a higher ceiling of maximal diuretic effect (i.e. efficacy) than other diuretics.

   (d) **False** Thiazide diuretics can aggravate pre-existing diabetes mellitus. One of the mechanisms proposed is the reduction of insulin secretion. Non thiazide diuretics might be used in this condition.

   (e) **True** Excitation of renal dopamine receptors causes renal vaso-dilatation, thereby increasing glomerular filtration and urine production. Dopamine may also increase cardiac output. Dopamine infusion is particularly used in toxaemic shock, when kidney function may be severely reduced. At high doses, dopamine causes vasoconstriction by stimulating α-adrenoceptors.

82 Frusemide:
   (a) causes potassium retention.
   (b) causes alkalosis.
   (c) is useful in the treatment of congestive heart failure.
   (d) is used for long term treatment of hypertension.
   (e) is not effective orally.

83 Spironolactone:
   (a) has a steroid structure.
   (b) is a partial agonist.
   (c) promotes Na^+ retention.
   (d) increases K^+ loss.
   (e) is a loop diuretic.

84 The following statements are true:
   (a) renin is an enzyme.
   (b) angiotensin I is converted to angiotensin II in the lungs.
   (c) angiotensin II can promote Na^+ retention.
   (d) angiotensin II is a potent vasodilator.
   (e) captopril is a competitive inhibitor of renin.

85 Inhibition of angiotensin converting enzyme (ACE):
   (a) prevents the conversion of renin to angiotensin I.
   (b) improves renal function.
   (c) is achieved with β-blockers.
   (d) can result in an increase in plasma K^+ concentration.
   (e) increases aldosterone production.

82 (a) **False**   As a result of the action of frusemide in the ascending loop of Henle, tubular fluid containing a large amount of Na^+ and Cl^- is delivered to the distal tubule, where Na^+ are actively reabsorbed in exchange for K^+ and H^+. There is therefore a loss of K^+.

(b) **True**   A metabolic alkalosis (an increase in the concentration of bicarbonate in the extracellular fluid) may arise from a reduction of extracellular volume if the mobilization of oedema fluid is rapid. In chronic therepy there is an increased output into the urine of H^+, which are exchanged for Na^+ – see (a). The latter are reabsorbed accompanied by a corresponding increase in HCO_3^-.

(c) **True**   An advantage with frusemide is its efficacy when the glomerular filtration rate is low, as in severe heart failure.

(d) **False**   It is usually only used for short term therapy.

(e) **False**   It can be given orally or intravenously.

83 (a) **True**   It is structurally similar to aldosterone.

(b) **False**   It is a competitive antagonist of aldosterone in the distal renal tubule.

(c) **False**   Aldosterone causes Na^+ reabsorption and K^+ loss in the distal tubule. Spironolactone antagonizes this effect.

(d) **False**   It conserves K^+. See (c).

(e) **False**   See (c).

84 (a) **True**   The decapeptide angiotensin I is formed from angiotensinogen by renin released from the kidney.

(b) **True**   The converting enzyme producing the octapeptide angiotensin II is mainly present in the lungs.

(c) **True**   Angiotensin II stimulates the synthesis and secretion of aldosterone by the adrenal cortex, which causes retention of Na^+.

(d) **False**   Angiotensin II is a vasoconstrictor, and on a molar basis is about 40 times more potent as a pressor agent than noradrenaline.

(e) **False**   Captopril inhibits the enzyme involved in converting angiotensin I to angiotensin II. Captopril is used to treat severe hypertension refractory to other treatment.

85 (a) **False**   Renin is an enzyme produced by the kidney which converts the globulin angiotensinogen into biologically inert angiotensin I. This is then converted by ACE into the vasoconstrictor angiotensin II. ACE inhibition prevents the conversion of angiotensin I to II.

(b) **False**   ACE inhibitors can precipitate renal failure; the mechanism by which they do so is not clearly understood.

(c) **False**   β-blockers reduce the release of renin from the juxtaglomerular cells. Captopril and enalapril are inhibitors of ACE.

(d) **True**   Angiotensin II stimulates the production of aldosterone which causes retention of Na^+, and K^+ excretion. ACE inhibition will reduce production of aldosterone and lessen K^+ excretion.

(e) **False**   See (d).

86 Osmotic diuretics:
(a) are filtered by the glomeruli.
(b) exert their effect mainly on the ascending loop of Henle.
(c) are useful in treating all causes of oedema.
(d) can reduce intracranial pressure.
(e) can be used in the treatment of glaucoma.

87 The acidity of gastric secretion can be modified in the following ways:
(a) decreased by propantheline.
(b) reduced by pentagastrin.
(c) increased by vagal stimulation.
(d) reduced by sodium bicarbonate.
(e) decreased by activation of histamine H_2-receptors.

88 Atropine-like substances.
(a) reduce the volume of gastric acid secretion.
(b) cause a substantial rise in the pH of gastric secretion.
(c) can be given in doses which specifically reduce the volume of gastric acid secretion.
(d) increase the rate of gastric emptying.
(e) decrease motility in the gastrointestinal tract.

89 The following statements about antacids are correct:
(a) aluminium hydroxide enhances the absorption of tetracycline.
(b) $NaHCO_3$ can cause systemic alkalosis.
(c) calcium carbonate causes systemic alkalosis.
(d) magnesium trisilicate can cause constipation.
(e) they are of no value in the treatment of duodenal ulcers.

86 (a) **True**
   (b) **False** Osmotic diuretics are filtered by the glomeruli but are only very poorly reabsorbed from renal tubular fluid. The main diuretic action is on the proximal tubule, which is a major site of water reabsorption.
   (c) **False** An infusion of an osmotic diuretic increases the plasma volume and is unsuitable for treating most causes of oedema, including cardiac failure.
   (d) **True** Mannitol and sucrose (administered intravenously) can be used in conditions such as head injury or brain tumour.
   (e) **True** By their osmotic effect in the blood, these substances reduce the formation of aqueous humour and can be used for the rapid reduction of intraocular pressure in acute glaucoma. They can also be used pre- and postoperatively in patients who require ocular surgery.

87 (a) **False** For whereas the volume of secretion may be decreased, the pH is not altered significantly.
   (b) **False** This substance, a synthetic derivative of gastrin, stimulates gastric acid secretion and is used as a test of gastric function.
   (c) **True**
   (d) **True** While the secretory process is unaffected, the acidity of stomach contents is decreased. It may produce systemic alkalosis.
   (e) **False** Activation of histamine H_2-receptors leads to an increase in gastric acid secretion.

88 (a) **True** But they do not significantly alter the pH.
   (b) **False** Even when given intravenously they do not do this.
   (c) **False** These compounds lack selectivity of action and cause unwanted effects, arising from their action on the parasympathetic nervous system; pirenzepine is selective for gastric muscarinic receptors.
   (d) **False** Their antimuscarinic action decreases gastric emptying and motility.
   (e) **True** They can cause constipation.

89 (a) **False** Tetracyclines chelate Al^{3+}, Ca^{2+} and Mg^{2+}, and the absorption of tetracylines from the gastrointestinal tract is reduced.
   (b) **True** Sodium bicarbonate can significantly alter the buffering capacity of plasma if taken in large doses.
   (c) **False** Carbonate ions are not well absorbed from the gastrointestinal tract.
   (d) **False** It tends to be laxative.
   (e) **False** They are valuable in the treatment of both gastric and duodenal ulceration. They produce relief of pain in most patients. The pH of the stomach contents is raised by neutralization of the acid, thereby reducing irritation. This is a contributory factor to the symptomatic relief provided by antacids.

90 Cimetidine:
    (a) reduces gastric acid secretion induced by pentagastrin.
    (b) blocks muscarinic receptors.
    (c) blocks histamine H_2-receptors.
    (d) raises the pH of gastric acid secretion.
    (e) reduces the volume of gastric acid secretion.

91 The treatment of gastric ulcers with carbenoxolone:
    (a) reduces the volume of gastric acid secretion.
    (b) causes a substantial rise in the pH of gastric secretion.
    (c) increases gastric emptying.
    (d) increases mucus production in the stomach.
    (e) may cause mineralocorticoid side-effects.

92 Constipation can be caused by:
    (a) propantheline.
    (b) ganglion-blocking drugs.
    (c) morphine.
    (d) magnesium sulphate.
    (e) methylcellulose.

93 The following statements about laxatives are correct.
    (a) the action of castor oil depends on its lubricant properties.
    (b) liquid paraffin acts by osmotically increasing the volume of gut contents.
    (c) sodium sulphate acts as an irritant purgative.
    (d) senna contains substances which on hydrolysis yield chemicals which
        increase colonic activity.
    (e) magnesium sulphate is well absorbed from the gastrointestinal tract.

90 (a) **True**   Gastric acid secretion induced by gastrin and muscarinic receptor agonists is also reduced by cimetidine. One possibility is that histamine is a common mediator of these agents with respect to effects on gastric acid secretion. Cimetidine is therefore a very efficient inhibitor of physiological secretion of gastric juice.

   (b) **False**   It is a selective competitive antagonist at histamine H_2-receptors which are involved in gastric secretion. However, it does reduce gastric secretion induced by muscarinic receptor agonists, e.g. bethanechol.

   (c) **True**   See (a).
   (d) **True**
   (e) **True**

91 (a) **False**   See (b).
   (b) **False**   Carbenoxolone does not reduce acid secretion, but it reduces the back-diffusion of H^+ into the gastric mucosa from the lumen of the stomach.

   (c) **False**
   (d) **True**   This may confer protection if the mucus adheres to the gastric mucosa. Carbenoxolone also prolongs the life-span of gastric epithelial cells.

   (e) **True** Na^+ retention, K^+ loss and hypertension can occur. The drug should not be given to patients receiving digitalis, the action of which is potentiated by hypokalaemia.

92 (a) **True**   This is a muscarinic receptor blocker which decreases gastro-intestinal motility.

   (b) **True**   Blockade of parasympathetic ganglia in the gut will cause constipation.

   (c) **True**   Morphine increases segmentation movements in the gut, causes constriction of sphincters and reduces peristalsis.

   (d) **False**   It is hardly absorbed from the gut and causes osmotic retention of water.

   (e) **False**   This is used as a bulk purgative. It takes up water, swelling to a colloid about 25 times its original volume.

93 (a) **False**   Castor oil is metabolized to ricinoleic acid which increases muscular contraction of the small intestine.

   (b) **False**   Liquid paraffin may have several actions, including softening the faeces and lubricating the large intestine.

   (c) **False**   Sulphate ions are poorly absorbed from the gut and thus cause water retention. Sodium sulphate is thus an osmotic purgative.

   (d) **True**   The main purgative constituents of senna are the anthraquinone derivatives, in particular the glycosides sennoside A and B. These glycosides are absorbed from the small intestine and hydrolysed in the liver to form aglycones, which increase colonic motility.

   (e) **False**   See 92(d).

94 The following drugs are effective in the treatment of motion sickness:
   (a) hyoscine.
   (b) propranolol.
   (c) promethazine.
   (d) cimetidine.
   (e) metoclopramide.

95 The following statements about therapy with iron are true:
   (a) iron deficiency can occur during pregnancy.
   (b) overdose of iron preparations can be treated with desferrioxamine.
   (c) ascorbic acid impairs the efficiency of iron absorption.
   (d) iron preparations should not be taken at the same time as tetracyclines.
   (e) gastrointestinal side-effects may limit the use of oral iron preparations.

96 Adrenocorticotrophic hormone (ACTH):
   (a) is synthesized in the adrenal cortex.
   (b) is ineffective when swallowed.
   (c) causes hypertrophy of the adrenal cortex.
   (d) secretion is suppressed by high blood levels of adrenaline.
   (e) is used as a diagnostic test for adrenal cortex function.

97 Hydrocortisone:
   (a) is synthesized in the adrenal medulla.
   (b) is effective when swallowed.
   (c) has purely mineralocorticoid activity.
   (d) can be antagonized by spironolactone.
   (e) very rarely causes side-effects when used for a long time.

94 (a) **True**   Muscarinic receptor blockade is effective in treating motion sickness.

  (b) **False**

  (c) **True**   Promethazine blocks histamine H_1-receptors but it is probable that its muscarinic receptor-blocking action is the important feature in this effect.

  (d) **False**

  (e) **False**   Whereas metoclopramide can reduce nausea and vomiting caused by drugs, it is not effective in reducing these symptoms of motion sickness.

95 (a) **True**   The fetus takes up to 600 mg iron from the mother during pregnancy, and dietary iron is seldom adequate to meet this demand.

  (b) **True**   This substance chelates iron and forms a non-toxic complex which is excreted in the urine. Desferrioxamine can be injected and, if given by gastric lavage, can also chelate iron in the gut, thus preventing further absorption.

  (c) **False**   Most iron in food is ferric iron and is absorbed mainly as ferrous iron. Reducing agents, such as ascorbic acid, increase the amount of ferrous iron in the gut.

  (d) **True**   Iron can be chelated by tetracyclines. The effectiveness of both preparations is reduced.

  (e) **True**   Nausea, gut pain and diarrhoea are reported side-effects of iron preparations, and patients may stop taking iron because of this. Other preparations can be tried but there is no convincing evidence that any one preparation is preferable to another.

96 (a) **False**   It is synthesized and released from the anterior pituitary. ACTH release is controlled by corticotrophin-releasing factors (CRF) synthesized in the hypothalamus and secreted into the local portal circulation. ACTH stimulates synthesis and release of corticosteroids from the adrenal cortex. There is a feedback control by corticosteroids which inhibit both ACTH and CRF production.

  (b) **True**   As it is a peptide, it must be injected intramuscularly. Tetracosactrin zinc injection is a slowly released depot injection.

  (c) **True**   Hypertrophy of the adrenal cortex can occur, in contrast to atrophy caused by corticosteroids.

  (d) **False**   ACTH secretion is suppressed by high blood levels of corticosteroids, not by adrenaline. See (a).

  (e) **True**   See (a).

97 (a) **False**   The precursor cortisone is synthesized in the adrenal cortex, and is converted to hydrocortisone in the liver.

  (b) **True**   Both cortisone and hydrocortisone can be given orally or parenterally.

  (c) **False**   It has both mineralocorticoid and glucocorticoid activity.

  (d) **True**   The mineralocorticoid actions of hydrocortisone (e.g. increased retention of Na^+ by the renal tubule) will be blocked by spironolactone. The glucocorticoid actions are not affected.

  (e) **False**   Numerous adverse effects occur during chronic administration (e.g. Cushing's syndrome), or following sudden withdrawal of any exogenously administered corticosteroid.

98 Corticosteroids with mainly glucocorticoid activity:
    (a) include prednisolone.
    (b) are free of actions in the CNS.
    (c) have anti-inflammatory actions.
    (d) do not suppress hypothalamic-pituitary-adrenal fuction.
    (e) include aldosterone.

99 Macrocortin:
    (a) is an endogenous glycoprotein.
    (b) synthesis is blocked by glucocorticoid.
    (c) is a derivative of hydrocortisone.
    (d) inhibits phospholipase A_2.
    (e) releases arachidonic acid.

100 Thyroxine:
    (a) is synthesized in the anterior pituitary.
    (b) is effective when swallowed.
    (c) is essential for normal growth.
    (d) synthesis is reduced by carbimazole.
    (e) increases oxygen consumption in most tissues.

98 (a) **True** Prednisolone is less potent than hydrocortisone with respect to mineralocorticoid activity, but is about four times more potent as a glucocorticoid and anti-inflammatory agent.

(b) **False** Depression, euphoria and psychotic responses can occur.

(c) **True** They are also used to suppress immune responses. For these effects, corticosteroids have to be given in high 'non-physiological' doses, when their metabolic effects become adverse reactions.

(d) **False** The high doses required for anti-inflammatory activity – see (c) – prevent release of corticotrophin-releasing hormone and thereby of corticotrophin, lack of which results in atrophy of the adrenal cortex. Sudden withdrawl of corticosteroids will leave the patient with little protection against stress.

(e) **False** Aldosterone has only mineralocorticoid activity, and its production is controlled mainly by plasma Na^+ and K^+ concentrations and plasma angiotensin II levels; corticotrophin has little effect on aldosterone production.

99 (a) **True** Macrocortin is so called because it is a large molecule originally isolated from rat macrophages and it mimics the effects of glucocorticoids.

(b) **False** Steroids with glucocorticoid activity are lipid-soluble molecules which enter cells and attach themselves to steroid receptors either in the cytoplasm or in the region of the nucleus of the cell. The steroid/receptor complex enters the nucleus and initiates protein synthesis by activating the appropriate genes to initiate formation of an appropriate messenger RNA. Macrocortin is one of the proteins synthesized as a result of the above process. Macrocortin then diffuses through the cytoplasm of the cell to its site of action.

(c) **False** Hydrocortisone and other steroids stimulate its synthesis and release.

(d) **True** Phospholipase A_2 is an enzyme which catalyses the release of arachidonic acid from membrane phospholipids. Inhibition of this enzyme reduces the release of arachidonic acid and so decreases the synthesis of prostaglandins and leucotrienes which are involved in inflammatory processes.

(e) **False** See (d).

100 (a) **False** Thyroid-stimulating hormone (TSH), which is synthesized in and released from the anterior pituitary, stimulates the release of thyroxine from the thyroid gland.

(b) **True** It is used to treat hypothyroid conditions (cretinism in children, myxoedema in adults) and simple goitre – though iodine may be the treatment of choice in the latter case.

(c) **True** It promotes normal growth and maturation, particularly of the CNS and skeleton.

(d) **True** Iodination of tyrosine is inhibited, and so thyroxine synthesis is reduced by carbimazole or propylthiouracil.

(e) **True** Metabolism is stimulated, the basal metabolic rate rises and protein synthesis increases.

101 Prolactin:
(a) is secreted from the anterior pituitary.
(b) secretion is inhibited by dopamine receptor agonists.
(c) secretion is increased by bromocriptine.
(d) inhibits the release of growth hormone.
(e) is used to treat infertility.

102 Oxytocin:
(a) is synthesized in the anterior pituitary.
(b) is ineffective when swallowed.
(c) decreases the tone and motility of the uterus.
(d) is potentiated by salbutamol.
(e) causes contraction of all smooth muscles.

103 The female oral contraceptive pill:
(a) contains androgens.
(b) can inhibit ovulation.
(c) frequently contains both oestrogen and progesterone.
(d) can increase the incidence of venous thrombosis.
(e) is free of effects on the CNS.

101 (a) **True**   It is a hormone which regulates lactation.

(b) **True**   Prolactin secretion is regulated by prolactin inhibitory hormone which is transported from the hypothalamus via the portal system to the anterior pituitary. Prolactin inhibitory hormone has been identified to be dopamine, and stimulation of dopamine receptors in the anterior pituitary leads to inhibition of release of prolactin.

(c) **False**   Bromocriptine is a dopamine receptor antagonist and is used to suppress lactation.

(d) **False**   Bromocriptine inhibits the release of growth hormone and is sometimes used in the treatment of acromegaly.

(e) **False**   It is the blockade of dopamine receptors resulting in excessive prolactin secretion which can lead to infertility. Prolactin in excess inhibits the release of gonadotrophic hormone releasing factors and this leads to infertility in males and females.

102 (a) **False**   Oxytocin and vasopressin (antidiuretic hormone) are synthesized in the anterior hypothalamic nuclei and transported along nerve fibres to the posterior pituitary, where they are stored and subsequently released. Oxytocin is reflexly released during parturition, following suckling, and by emotion stimuli.

(b) **True**   It is absorbed from the buccal mucosa, but it is most frequently given in an intravenous infusion.

(c) **False**   It is used to induce or speed labour, when it increases tone and motility of the uterus. Uterine smooth muscle becomes much more sensitive to oxytocin at term.

(d) **False**   Salbutamol causes relaxation of the uterus, and it is used to prevent premature labour.

(e) **False**   Uterine smooth muscle contracts in response to oxytocin. Vascular smooth muscle is usually relaxed by oxytocin and this can cause hypotension. However, it must be used with caution as vasoconstriction and hypertension (possibly a reflex stress response) can occur.

103 (a) **False**

(b) **True**

(c) **True**

(d) **True**

(e) **False**

104 Insulin:
   (a) is synthesized in the α-cells of the islets of Langerhans in the pancreas.
   (b) is effective orally when combined with zinc.
   (c) increases the permeability of cells to glucose.
   (d) has actions opposite to glucagon.
   (e) is potentiated by non-selective β-adrenoceptor blockers.

105 Glucagon:
   (a) is synthesized in the β-cells of the islets of Langerhans in the pancreas.
   (b) can be administered by injection.
   (c) increases the synthesis and storage of glycogen in the liver.
   (d) is antagonized by adrenaline in its effects on the blood sugar.
   (e) is used in the treatment of acute hypoglycaemic coma.

106 α-methyl DOPA:
   (a) causes hypotension by acting as an inhibitor of DOPA decarboxylase.
   (b) is converted into a false transmitter.
   (c) hypotension could be reversed by carbidopa.
   (d) can cause confusion and depression.
   (e) often causes orthostatic hypotension.

104 (a) **False** It is synthesized in and released from the β-cells of the islets of Langerhans.

(b) **False** As insulin is a peptide it cannot be taken orally. The various preparations include: soluble insulin (fast acting, short duration of action); insulin zinc suspension (longer acting, slower onset of action); crystalline insulin zinc suspension (long duration of action). Soluble insulin can be given intravenously, intramuscularly or subcutaneously; other insulins are usually given subcutaneously.

(c) **True** Glucose uptake into muscle and fat tissue is increased; it is there converted into glycogen and fat respectively.

(d) **True** See 105.

(e) **True** These compounds will decrease the release of glucose from the liver mediated by sympathetic stimulation which occurs during hypoglycaemia. As insulin causes a hypoglycaemic response, a potentiation of this effect occurs. Adrenergic neurone blockers also potentiate insulin.

105 (a) **False** It is synthesized in and released from the α-cells of the islets of Langerhans in response to hypoglyaemia.

(b) **True** It has actions which oppose those of insulin. It is used to treat hypoglycaemic coma induced by insulin overdose. Glucose may also be necessary in such circumstances, either intravenously (if the person is unconscious) or by mouth.

(c) **False** Its major action is glycogenolysis in the liver and release of glucose.

(d) **False** Adrenaline causes glycogenolysis in both liver and muscle, and brings about an increase in blood glucose concentration.

(e) **True** Glucagon and/or glucose are treatments of choice.

106 (a) **False** α-methyl DOPA is potent inhibitor of DOPA decarboxylase *in vitro*. To be effective, α-methyl DOPA must be decarboxylated to α-methyl dopamine and then α-methyl noradrenaline in the CNS, where α-methyl noradrenaline acts as a false transmitter at α_2-adrenoceptors. This results in a decrease in peripheral sympathetic tone.

(b) **True** See (a).

(c) **False** Carbidopa does not penetrate into the CNS, thus it would not interfere with the decarboxylation of α-methyl DOPA.

(d) **True** Confusion and depression are common side-effects of treatment with α-methyl DOPA, occurring more frequently in the elderly.

(e) **False** The baroceptor reflex is less likely to be impaired by this drug than by hypotensive agents such as adrenergic neurone blockers.

107 The following drug interactions may occur in persons treated with
     monoamine oxidase (MAO) inhibitors:
     (a) hypertension after administration of L-DOPA.
     (b) antagonism of the hypotensive actions of guanethidine.
     (c) a hypotensive response following ingestion of foods containing tyramine.
     (d) a decreased response to tolbutamide.
     (e) potentiation and prolongation of the action of pethidine.

108 Tricyclic antidepressants such as imipramine:
     (a) are free of adverse effects on the heart.
     (b) can cause convulsions.
     (c) are routinely used in conjunction with MAO inhibitors in the treatment of
         endogenous depression.
     (d) can cause dry mouth and blurred vision.
     (e) can cause postural hypotension.

109 Methylxanthines:
     (a) can have an arousing effect in the CNS.
     (b) can increase intracellular levels of cyclic AMP.
     (c) compete for adenosine-binding sites.
     (d) include aminophylline which causes bronchodilatation.
     (e) decrease calcium entry into intracellular stores.

110 Cocaine:
     (a) blocks the re-uptake of noradrenaline into all noradrenergic neurones.
     (b) can cause cardiac dysrhythmias.
     (c) has local anaesthetic properties.
     (d) is used as an antidepressant.
     (e) can cause euphoria.

107 (a) **True**   L-DOPA is decarboxylated to dopamine in many tissues (e.g. gut, liver). Normally, when MAO is active, the dopamine would be inactivated within these tissues. When MAO is inhibited, dopamine enters the systemic circulation, where it has a sympathomimetic effect at both α- and β-adrenoceptors.

(b) **False**   A greater hypotension may result, as MAO inhibitors have themselves some hypotensive actions.

(c) **False**   A hypertensive response is most likely. Tyramine is an indirectly acting sympathomimetic amine (see Question 30) which is usually destroyed in the gut and liver by MAO.

(d) **False**   A potentiation of the hypoglycaemic response to tolbutamide may occur, as MAO inhibitors inhibit enzymes other than the MAO thus slowing metabolism of tolbutamide.

(e) **True**   Possibly by a mechanism similar to that in (d). Examples of MAO inhibitors are iproniazid, phenelzine and tranylcypromine.

108 (a) **False**   Inhibition of noradrenaline uptake can lead to tachycardia and cardiac dysrhythmias, as these drugs not only block amine uptake in the CNS, but also in the sympathetic nervous system.

(b) **True**   Children are particularly liable to this adverse effect.

(c) **False**   Severe adverse effects such as confusion, high body temperature, coma and death have been reported when these two groups of antidepressants have been used at the same time.

(d) **True**   Tricylic antidepressants have central and peripheral antimuscarinic actions. Constipation, urinary retention and tachycardia are other adverse effects. Mianserin, iprindole and nomifensine are antidepressants which have weaker anti-muscarinic side-effects.

(e) **True**   This has been attributed to an α_1-adrenoceptor blocking action. Mianserin, iprindole and nomifensine are less liable to cause such problems.

109 (a) **True**   The methylxanthines, caffeine, theophylline, aminophylline and theobromine, can all cause arousal and wakefulness if they enter the CNS.

(b) **True**   At concentrations higher than those usually encountered *in vivo*, methylxanthines can inhibit phosphodiesterases – enzymes which inactivate cyclic AMP. When these enzymes are inhibited, the level of cyclic AMP is increased.

(c) **True**   While it is not clear whether adenosine, or adenosine compounds, act as neurotransmitters, they are potent agonists in many tissues. Methylxanthines have been shown to be competitive antagonists of adenosine in some tissues, and in ligand-binding studies using cell membrane preparations.

(d) **True**   Aminophylline is used in the treatment of bronchial asthma.

(e) **True**   This action may contribute to some of the effects of methylxanthines, for example the cardiac stimulant effect which can cause dysrhythmias.

110 (a) **True**

(b) **True**

(c) **True**   It is now rarely used for this purpose, as other less toxic local anaesthetics are available.

(d) **False**

(e) **True**   Higher doses can lead to psychotic behaviour.

111 The following act as dopamine-receptor agonists:
   (a) metoclopramide.
   (b) fluphenazine decanoate.
   (c) bromocryptine.
   (d) benztropine.
   (e) amantidine.

112 Blockade of dopamine receptors:
   (a) can be an effective treatment for psychotic conditions.
   (b) occurs with haloperidol.
   (c) can lead to infertility.
   (d) can cause a Parkinsonian syndrome.
   (e) is an effective treatment of depression.

113 Vomiting can be caused by:
   (a) blockade of dopamine receptors in the chemoreceptor trigger zone.
   (b) metoclopramide.
   (c) ipecacuanha.
   (d) 5-HT3 antagonists.
   (e) naloxone.

111 (a) **False**   Metoclopramide selectively blocks dopamine receptors associated with drug-induced nausea and emesis, and is used as an antiemetic. It is not effective in the treatment of motion sickness.

(b) **False**   Fluphenazine decanoate is a sustained-release preparation used in the treatment of schizophrenia. Fluphenazine acts as a dopamine-receptor blocker.

(c) **True**   Bromocryptine is a direct dopamine-receptor agonist. It is used in the treatment of prolactin-induced infertility where it mimics the actions of dopamine. It is also used in the treatment of acromegaly, where it has been suggested that dopamine is underactive as an inhibitor of growth-hormone release. It is used to treat Parkinson's disease.

(d) **False**   Benztropine inhibits the re-uptake of dopamine into dopaminergic terminals. It has antimuscarinic actions. It is used in the treatment of Parkinson's disease.

(e) **True**   This is an indirectly acting dopamine-receptor agonist. It is used in Parkinson's disease and works by releasing dopamine from intact dopaminergic neurones.

112 (a) **True**   The dopamine theory of psychosis states that there may be overactivity of certain dopaminergic pathways. Dopamine – receptor blockers such as the phenothiazines (chlorpromazine, fluphenazine) and butyrophenones (haloperidol) have antipsychotic activity.

(b) **True**

(c) **True**   Dopamine is believed to be prolactin inhibitory factor (PIF), which inhibits the release of prolactin from the anterior pituitary. If dopamine receptors are blocked, uncontrolled release of prolactin occurs. This leads to inhibition (of release) of gonadotrophic hormone-releasing factors, which causes infertility in females and males.

(d) **True**   This is a major side-effect of antipsychotic drugs.

(e) **False**

113 (a) **False**   Stimulation of dopamine receptors in the chemoreceptor trigger zone causes vomiting.

(b) **False**   Metoclopramide blocks dopamine receptors and can prevent vomiting induced by dopamine agonists.

(c) **True**   Ipecacuanha and cardiac glycosides cause vomiting by acting both in the chemoreceptor trigger zone and in the gastrointestinal tract.

(d) **False**   5-HT3 antagonists, for example odansetron, are highly effective antiemetics. They are particularly effective in the treatment of vomiting caused by chemotherapy and radiotherapy. Odansetron is a competitive antagonist of 5-HT3 receptors which are found both in the gastrointestinal tract and in the area postrema of the brain which contains the chemoreceptor trigger zone. Inhibition of chemoreceptor mechanisms either in the central nervous system or in the gut can be effective at inhibiting vomiting.

(e) **False**   Morphine or apomorphine but not the morphine antagonist naloxone, cause vomiting.

114 Dopa decarboxylase:
  (a) is present in adrenergic nerve fibres.
  (b) catalyses the conversion of tryptophan to tyramine.
  (c) catalyses the conversion of 5-hydroxtryptophan to serotonin.
  (d) converts levodopa to dopamine.
  (e) is inhibited by benserazide.

115 When L-DOPA is used in the treatment of Parkinson's disease it:
  (a) has useful anti-emetic activity.
  (b) may be combined with carbidopa to reduce metabolism of L-DOPA
      outside the brain.
  (c) is converted to a false transmitter.
  (d) can cause psychotic behaviour.
  (e) is actively taken up by dopaminergic neurones in the CNS.

116 The following drugs, by affecting dopaminergic mechanisms, can have the
     actions indicated:
  (a) neuroleptics can induce akathesia.
  (b) reserpine can alleviate the symptoms of Parkinson's disease.
  (c) chlorpromazine can bring about tardive dyskinesias.
  (d) chlorpromazine can be used to treat tardive dyskinesias.
  (e) mazindol has anorectic activity.

114 (a) **True** It is found in all cells in the body. Dopa decarboxylase is a trivial name for the enzyme L aromatic aminoacid decarboxylase.

(b) **False** Dopa decarboxylase catalyses the converion of tryptophan to tryptamine.

(c) **True**

(d) **True**

(e) **True** Benserazide is not very lipid soluble, so it does not penetrate the blood-brain barrier and is used in Parkinson's disease with L-DOPA to prevent the peripheral decarboxylation of the latter. Carbidopa is another peripheral dopa decarboxylase inhibitor used for the same purposes as benserazide. Dopa decarboxylase inhibitors which penetrate the blood-brain barrier are of experimental interest only.

115 (a) **False** Nausea and vomiting may limit the therapeutic usefulness of L-DOPA. Tolerance to this action of L-DOPA does develop. and this effect can be reduced by:
(i) increasing the dose of L-DOPA gradually.
(ii) taking L-DOPA with food, and
(iii) taking carbidopa – see (b).

(b) **True** Carbidopa (L-α-methyl DOPA hydrazine) is an inhibitor of DOPA decarboxylase, and does not cross the blood-brain barrier.

(c) **False** L-DOPA is converted to the real transmitter dopramine.

(d) **True** L-DOPA therapy can cause psychotic reactions, more commonly in those with a previous history of psychosis.

(e) **True** It is also taken up by glial cells in the CNS, but diffuses out of them as they do not have storage mechanisms. It has been suggested that glial cells are an important site of decarboxylation in Parkinson's disease, when the number of dopaminergic neurones and terminals are reduced.

116 (a) **True** This can be defined as an inability to remain still. It is a motor restlessness, and may be the result of partial agonist activity at dopamine receptors of some neuroleptics (antipsychotic drugs). It generally occurs during the early stages of drug treatment.

(b) **False** Reserpine will induce a Parkinsonian syndrome, or make existing Parkinson's disease worse.

(c) **True** Following prolonged use (months or years) of neuroleptics, abnormal movements, particularly of the mouth, tongue, and face, can occur. This may be due to development of increased sensitivity of dopamine receptors to compensate for prolonged block. Tardive dyskinesias can be treated by increasing the dose of neuroleptic.

(d) **True**

(e) **True** Mazindol causes dopamine release and inhibits its re-uptake into neurones. There is evidence that excitation of dopamine receptors in the hypothalamus is a mechanism involved in anorexia (suppression of appetite).

117 Chlorpromazine:
  (a) is used to treat Parkinson's disease.
  (b) causes a dry mouth.
  (c) causes urinary retention.
  (d) causes gynaecomastia.
  (e) is a useful appetite suppressant.

118 Major tranquillizers:
  (a) are used as hypnotics.
  (b) are drugs such as barbiturates and benzodiazepines.
  (c) include the phenothiazines and butyrophenones.
  (d) are used in the treatment of psychotic disorders.
  (e) frequently have dopamine-receptor blocking properties.

119 5-HT:
  (a) storage is disrupted by reserpine.
  (b) concentration in nerves is increased by MAO inhibitors.
  (c) can cause increased gastrointestinal motility.
  (d) stored in enterochromaffin cells has a neurotransmitter role.
  (e) re-uptake into neurones is unaffected by clomipramine.

120 The following drugs affect 5-HT mechanisms in the ways indicated:
  (a) L-tryptophan blocks the synthesis of 5-HT.
  (b) methysergide is a 5-HT receptor agonist.
  (c) lysergic acid diethylamide (LSD) is a 5-HT receptor blocker.
  (d) fenfluramine can release 5-HT.
  (e) cyproheptadine can block 5-HT receptors.

121 The following are amino-acid neurotransmitters which decrease neural activity:
  (a) glycine.
  (b) glutamic acid.
  (c) gamma-amino butyric acid (GABA).
  (d) leucine enkephalin.
  (e) tyrosine.

117 (a) **False** Chlorpromazine blocks dopamine receptors and causes extrapyramidal symptoms as seen in Parkinson's disease.

   (b) **True** Chlorpromazine blocks muscarinic receptors and has weak anticholinergic actions.

   (c) **True** See (b).

   (d) **True** Pituitary secretion of prolactin is under inhibitory control from the hypothalamus by prolactin-inhibitory hormone (PIH)-dopamine. Chlorpromazine blocks dopamine receptors and so prolactin secretion increases. Prolactin inhibits the release of gonadotrophic-hormone-releasing hormone so less testosterone is secreted and female sex characteristics such as gynaecomastia occur in males.

   (e) **False** Chlorpromazine causes a gain in weight and an increase in appetite.

118 (a) **False** Minor tranquillizers are used for this purpose. Major tranquillizers are used in the treatment of psychoses.

   (b) **False** These compounds are minor tranquillizers.

   (c) **True** Chlorpromazine and fluphenazine are phenothiazines; halperidol is a butyrophenone.

   (d) **True**

   (e) **True**

119 (a) **True** Reserpine disrupts the storage of all monoamines.

   (b) **True** Monoamine oxidase metabolizes 5-HT to 5-hydroxy-indole acetic acid.

   (c) **True** This may be the explanation for diarrhoea following treatment with fenfluramine or reserpine.

   (d) **False** Only 5-HT stored in nerves has a neurotransmitter role Enterochromaffin cells are not neurones.

   (e) **False** Clomipramine, a tricylic antidepressant, blocks 5-HT re-uptake.

120 (a) **False** L-tryptophan is the precursor of 5-HT.

   (b) **False** It is a 5-HT receptor blocker.

   (c) **True**

   (d) **True** Fenfluramine is used as an anorectic, which both releases 5-HT and blocks its neuronal re-uptake.

   (e) **True** It has been used to stimulate appetite in children, thus it may have an action which is the opposite of fenfluramine. It can reduce intestinal hypermotility caused by 5-HT release. Additionally, it blocks histamine H_1-receptors.

121 (a) **True** Glycine is an inhibitory neurotransmitter in the spinal cord.

   (b) **False** It increases neuronal activity.

   (c) **True**

   (d) **False** Leucine enkephalin is a peptide neurotransmitter.

   (e) **False** Tyrosine, a precursor of dopamine, noradrenaline and adrenaline, is an amino acid, but not a neurotransmitter.

122 Gamma-amino butyric acid (GABA):
   (a) is found in high concentrations in the basal ganglia.
   (b) concentrations in the basal ganglia are abnormally low in Huntingdon's chorea.
   (c) receptors are sensitive to the activity of benzodiazepines.
   (d) metabolism is inhibited by sodium valproate.
   (e) receptor blockers have anticonvulsant activity.

123 Lithium:
   (a) is used as an anxiolytic.
   (b) has a large therapeutic/toxic ratio.
   (c) is best given at 4 hourly intervals.
   (d) is more toxic in Na^+ depleted patients.
   (e) toxicity can be reversed by a thiazide diuretic.

124 The following statements about benzodiazepines are true:
   (a) they lack anxiolytic activity.
   (b) they are used as hypnotics.
   (c) they have anticonvulsant actions.
   (d) they are effective antidepressants.
   (e) they are free of the risk of dependence.

122 (a) **True**
   (b) **True**   As GABA acts as an inhibitory neurotransmitter in the basal ganglia, its loss at these sites in Huntingdon's chorea may be causally linked with the abnormal movements which occur in this condition.
   (c) **True**   It has been suggested that benzodiazepines act as modulators of GABA receptor sensitivity. Evidence from ligand-binding studies suggested that they increase the affinity of GABA binding sites for GABA. The nature of the endogenous ligand which binds to the benzodiazepine receptor is not known.
   (d) **True**   Sodium valproate is an inhibitor of GABA transaminase. It is not clear whether this action contributes to its anti-convulsant property.
   (e) **False**   GABA-receptor blockers such as bicuculline and picrotoxin are convulsants.

123 (a) **False**   Lithium is used in the treatment of manic depressive psychosis and occasionally in the treatment of unipolar depressive illness.
   (b) **False**   Therefore lithium should not be prescribed unless facilities are available for monitoring plasma concentrations.
   (c) **False**   The half-life of lithium is 15–30 hours and it is usually given 12 hourly to avoid large fluctuations in plasma concentration since the therapeutic/toxic ratio is small. The therapeutic range of lithium concentration in plasma is between 0.6 to 1.2 millimoles lithium per litre. Toxic symptoms occur if the plasma concentration increases to 1.5 millimoles lithium per litre. Toxic effects include ataxia, slurred speech, nystagmus, tremor, convulsions and possibly death. Weight gain due to fluid retention occurs at therapeutic concentrations of lithium.
   (d) **True**   Lithium is eliminated in the urine. It is filtered at the glomerulus and reabsorbed in the renal tubule along with sodium. In sodium depletion (e.g. after giving a diuretic) lithium is retained in the body and toxicity can be precipitated.
   (e) **False**   Thiazide diuretics increase sodium excretion thus they will increase lithium toxicity.

124 (a) **False**   Their anxiolytic activity (i.e. the reduction of fearfulness) is one of their valuable properties.
   (b) **True**
   (c) **True**   Diazepam and clonazepam can be given intravenously to control status epilepticus, and clonazepam is used in the treatment of grand mal epilepsy.
   (d) **False**
   (e) **False**   Whereas it is not clearly established that physical dependence occurs, psychological dependence is common.

125 Temazepam:
 (a) produces inactive metabolites.
 (b) increases rapid eye movement (REM) sleep.
 (c) is a potent enzyme inducer.
 (d) causes less hangover than nitrazepam.
 (e) causes rebound insomnia.

126 The following can occur following prolonged use of barbiturates:
 (a) tolerance to the actions of other hypnotics.
 (b) bleeding by displacing warfarin from plasma protein-binding sites.
 (c) abnormally rapid metabolism of oestrogens.
 (d) status epilepticus on withdrawal of barbiturate.
 (e) tolerance to a similar degree to both the hypnotic and respiratory depressant actions.

127 The following barbiturates are commonly used for the purposes indicated:
 (a) thiopentone – as an anxiolytic.
 (b) methohexitone – for the relief of pain.
 (c) phenobarbitone – in status epilepticus.
 (d) phenobarbitone – in long-term therapy of epilepsy.
 (e) pentobarbitone – to induce general anaesthesia.

125 (a) **True** In contrast to diazepam which has active metabolites.
   (b) **False** Benzodiazepines suppress REM sleep; no hypnotic induces natural sleep.
   (c) **False** Benzodiazepines induce enzymes to a minimal extent.
   (d) **True** The hangover-inducing effect of nitrazepam taken at bedtime may carry over into the afternoon of the following day. Temazepam has little or no hangover effect compared to nitrazepam.
   (e) **True** Benzodiazepines such as temazepam with a relatively short plasma half-life (6–8 hours) are more likely to cause rebound insomnia. Rebound insomnia is the inability to sleep upon waking some 5–6 hours after taking temazepam. It has been suggested that rebound insomnia is a form of withdrawal symptom from the effects of the short-acting benzodiazepines. Benzodiazepines with a long plasma half-life do not cause this form of insomnia (because high plasma concentrations of the drug are still present 6–8 hours after taking the drug). Dependence on all types of benzodiazepines (and other drugs used as hypnotics) occurs, and is characterized by difficulty in getting to sleep if the drug is not taken. This indicates that a form of physical dependence occurs when these drugs are taken regularly.

126 (a) **True** Cross-tolerance occurs to other hypnotics, e.g. chloral hydrate, glutethimide, whereby the hypnotic effect of these compounds decreases, partly due to induction of hepatic enzymes by barbiturates.
   (b) **False** Whereas barbiturates may displace some warfarin from plasma protein, this does not appear to be sufficient to cause problems in practice. But see 78(e).
   (c) **True** This may account for the occasional failure of oral contraceptives. Barbiturates induce (i.e. increase the amount of) liver microsomal enzymes which metabolize drugs, including oestrogens, barbiturates themselves, and warfarin.
   (d) **True** Rapid withdrawal of anticonvulsant is one of the most common causes of status epilepticus.
   (e) **False** While marked tolerance occurs to the hypnotic effects, tolerance occurs to a lesser extent to the respiratory depressant effect of barbiturates.

127 (a) **False** It is very lipid soluble and is used as an intravenous anesthetic.
   (b) **False** Barbiturates do not have analgesic actions.
   (c) **False** Phenobarbitone is used in long-term management of grand mal epilepsy. It is not very lipid soluble and is only slowly absorbed into the CNS, even after intravenous injection.
   (d) **True**
   (e) **False** Pentobarbitone has been used as an anxiolytic and hypnotic; it is not as lipid soluble as thiopentone.

128 The following statements are true.
   (a) phenytoin can induce its own metabolism.
   (b) primidone is metabolized to phenobarbitone.
   (c) sodium valproate is effective in all forms of epilepsy.
   (d) phenytoin can cause gum hyperplasia and acne.
   (e) ethosuximide is used in the treatment of petit mal epilepsy.

129 The following are used in the treatment of grand mal epilepsy:
   (a) phenytoin.
   (b) phenobarbitone.
   (c) nikethamide.
   (d) diazepam.
   (e) primidone.

130 The following drugs can cause convulsions.
   (a) doxapram.
   (b) strychnine.
   (c) tricyclic antidepressants.
   (d) methohexitone.
   (e) picrotoxin.

131 Blockade of muscarinic receptors in the CNS:
   (a) by hyoscine leads to agitation and excitement.
   (b) causes nausea and vomiting.
   (c) by hyoscine can impair short-term memory.
   (d) by atropine may be reversed by physostigmine.
   (e) by benztropine can decrease tremor in Parkinson's disease.

132 Morphine:
   (a) mimics the actions of enkephalins.
   (b) does not cause dependence.
   (c) can cause constipation.
   (d) acts as a partial agonist.
   (e) is only administered orally.

128 (a) **True** Phenytoin, phenobarbitone and primidone all induce liver microsomal enzymes which metabolize these compounds to biologically less active products.

(b) **True** It is believed that most of the anticonvulsant effect of primidone is caused by the metabolite phenobarbitone, but primidone itself, and other metabolites may also have anticonvulsant actions.

(c) **True**

(d) **True** These are among the common adverse effects. Others include nausea, headache and insomnia. Loss of coordination and slurred speech occur with overdose.

(e) **True** Ethosuximide is not effective against grand mal seizures.

129 (a) **True**

(b) **True**

(c) **False** This is an analeptic, which is occasionally used as a respiratory stimulant. However, it is a general CNS stimulant and can cause convulsions.

(d) **False** It causes unacceptable sedation at doses which will be effective in grand mal epilepsy.

(e) **True**

130 (a) **True** It is used as respiratory stimulant, but the dose needed to stimulate respiration is close to that which causes convulsions (i.e. a low therapeutic ratio).

(b) **True** This is a blocker at glycine receptors in the spinal cord, where glycine is an inhibitory transmitter.

(c) **True** This can occur when they are used at conventional therapeutic doses in susceptible adults (the risk is increased in people with epilepsy). Children appear to be more susceptible to this effect.

(d) **True**

(e) **True** This is an antagonist at GABA-A receptors in the spinal cord.

131 (a) **False** Hyoscine tends to cause sedation; atropine, however, does cause agitation and excitement.

(b) **False** Hyoscine is used to prevent travel sickness. Other drugs with antimuscarinic actions have similar effects.

(c) **True** Cholinergic mechanisms appear to be vital for short-term memory. In Alzheimer's disease (pre-senile dementia in which loss of short-term memory is a major symptom), there is a decreased ability to synthesize acetylcholine in the CNS because of deficiencies of choline acetyl transferase.

(d) **True** Physostigmine, an inhibitor of acetylcholinesterase, enters the CNS.

(e) **True** Anticholinergic drugs such as hyoscine were the first effective treatment for Parkinson's disease. They do not improve hypokinesia and only reduce the tremor.

132 (a) **True**

(b) **False** It causes both physical and physiological dependence.

(c) **True**

(d) **False**

(e) **False** It is also injected intramuscularly.

133 β-endorphin is:
    (a) a peptide.
    (b) a neurotransmitter.
    (c) present in the pituitary.
    (d) an opiate-receptor antagonist.
    (e) an analgesic.

134 H_1-receptor blockers:
    (a) have an arousing action in the CNS.
    (b) are used as anti-emetics.
    (c) include chlorpromazine.
    (d) may have muscarinic receptor-blocking actions.
    (e) prevent histamine-induced gastric secretion.

135 Codeine:
    (a) occurs in opium.
    (b) frequently causes diarrhoea.
    (c) is used to treat nausea caused by morphine.
    (d) is equipotent to morphine.
    (e) depresses the cough reflex.

136 Indicate whether the following statements are correct:
    (a) naxloxone will precipitate withdrawal symptoms in a morphine addict.
    (b) naloxone is useful in treating barbiturate-induced respiratory depression.
    (c) pethidine is a useful cough suppressant.
    (d) pethidine constricts the pupil.
    (e) nalorphine is a partial agonist.

133 (a) **True** β-endorphin is an endogenous opioid peptide derived from β-lipotropin, a fat-mobilizing hormone of the pituitary. β-endorphin has analgesic and other pharmacological actions similar to morphine.

   (b) **True** β-endorphine is the most potent endogenous agonist at μ-opiate receptors. β-endorphin-like immunoactivity is found on neurones in the central nervous system, and this is taken to indicate that β-endorphin has a neurotransmitter function in addition to any hormonal functions.

   (c) **True** See (a).

   (d) **False** β-endorphin is the most potent μ-opioid receptor agonist known. Naloxone has a higher affinity for μ-opioid receptors than for δ or κ opioid receptors.

   (e) **True** It is not used therapeutically for this purpose; it also causes respiratory depression, tolerance and withdrawal symptoms, suggesting that it can cause physical dependence.

134 (a) **False** Histamine H_1-receptor blockers generally cause drowsiness and sedation, and can cause sleep.

   (b) **True** Their antimuscarinic property may be responsible for the anti-emetic action which is particularly effective in the treatment of motion sickness.

   (c) **True** Chlorpromazine blocks histamine H_1, muscarinic, dopamine and α-adrenoceptors. It is less potent than selective blockers at these sites.

   (d) **True** See (b).

   (e) **False** Histamine H_2-blockers do this.

135 (a) **True**

   (b) **False** Codeine causes spasm of intestinal muscle and decreases peristalsis. It is used to decrease gastrointestinal motility.

   (c) **False** Nausea is an unwanted effect of codeine.

   (d) **False** Codeine has approximately one-tenth the potency of morphine.

   (e) **True**

136 (a) **True** Naloxone is a competitive antagonist of morphine at opiate receptors.

   (b) **False** Naloxone acts only at opiate receptors. Barbiturates depress respiration by acting at sites other than opiate receptors. and there are no competitive antagonists for barbiturates.

   (c) **False**

   (d) **False** Pethidine has some atropine-like activity and in overdose is likely to dilate the pupil.

   (e) **True** It stimulates opiate receptors before blocking them. With the availability of naloxone it has ceased to be the drug of choice in reversing the toxic effects of opiates, as the agonist action can initially (and possibly fatally) depress respiration further.

137 The following statements are true:
    (a) tolerance to, and dependence on, ethanol do not occur.
    (b) methanol is more rapidly metabolized than ethanol.
    (c) ethanol can be given to reduce the toxic actions of methanol.
    (d) ethanol is a clinically used diuretic.
    (e) ethanol metabolism is accelerated by disulfiram.

138 Hallucinations can occur with the following drugs:
    (a) tetrahydrocannabinol.
    (b) 2-bromolysergide.
    (c) pentazocine.
    (d) naloxone.
    (e) ethanol.

139 The following statement(s) about general anaesthetics are correct:
    (a) enflurane commonly causes liver disfunction.
    (b) halothane should not be used in patients requiring repeated anaesthesia.
    (c) general anaesthetics cause respiratory depression.
    (d) ketamine has useful analgesic properties.
    (e) the action of thiopentone is terminated by redistribution from plasma to well-vascularized tissues.

140 Nitrous oxide:
    (a) can be used, with oxygen, as a carrier gas for halothane.
    (b) has poor analgesic properties.
    (c) forms a vapour which is explosive.
    (d) sensitizes the heart to the actions of catecholamines.
    (e) is an effective agent for inducing anaesthesia.

141 Halothane is a general anaesthetic which:
    (a) is inflammable.
    (b) irritates mucous membranes.
    (c) can cause liver damage.
    (d) can sensitize the heart to the actions of catecholamines.
    (e) can cause vasomotor and respiratory depression.

137 (a) **False**   Both tolerance (a decreased response to the same dose of drug) and dependence (the occurrence of withdrawal symptoms when the drug is no longer taken) occur after prolonged use of ethanol.

(b) **False**   Metabolism of methanol is much slower than that of ethanol.

(c) **True**   Ethanol and methanol share the same biochemical pathway of metabolism. Ethanol can reduce the rate of metabolism of methanol.

(d) **False**   It inhibits the secretion of ADH, which results in less water being absorbed in the collecting ducts. This diuresis is only of water, there is no extra loss of Na^+, which is what is sought in a therapeutically useful diuretic.

(e) **False**   Disulfiram slows ethanol metabolism by inhibiting aldehyde dehydrogenase. The abnormally high levels of acetaldehyde which occur in such circumstances lead to a malaise which the person associates with drinking ethanol, and which discourages him from taking any more ethanol.

138 (a) **True**   This is one of the active constituents of cannabis.

(b) **False**   Unlike lysergide (LSD), this derivative of LSD has no reported hallucinogenic activity.

(c) **True**   This is an analgesic about three to four times less potent than morphine.

(d) **False**   This is a competitive antagonist at opiate receptors.

(e) **True**   Delirium trements can occur during alochol withdrawal in dependent subjects.

139 (a) **False**   Halothane can cause this problem if a person is repeatedly exposed to it. Enflurane may be preferred if a patient has to be anaesthetized on several occasions.

(b) **True**   See (a).

(c) **True**   If this occurs, pCO_2 can rise and cause cardiac dysrhythmias.

(d) **True**   Ketamine is given parenterally, and analgesia occurs at subanaesthetic doses.

(e) **True**

140 (a) **True**   This combines the analgesia caused by nitrous oxide with the more potent anaesthetic effect of halothane.

(b) **False**   As a 50:50 mixture with oxygen (Entonox), nitrous oxide is used as an analgesic, especially in obstetrics.

(c) **False**   Nitrous oxide will support combustion, but does not form explosive mixtures with air.

(d) **False**

(e) **False**   It is difficult to induce anaesthesia with nitrous oxide yet at the same time maintain adequate oxygenation. It is therefore not used for this purpose.

141 (a) **False**

(b) **False**

(c) **True**   This appears to be a form of hypersensitivity. It is most common after repeated exposure to halothane.

(d) **True**   This is an adverse effect of all halogenated anaesthetics and can cause dysrhythmias.

(e) **True**   Low blood pressure and respiratory arrest can occur.

142 Thiopentone:
    (a) is a highly lipid-soluble barbiturate.
    (b) is used intravenously to induce anaesthesia.
    (c) has its anaesthetic action terminated by metabolism to an inactive compound.
    (d) has good analgesic properties.
    (e) can cause convulsive movements.

143 The mechanisms of action of the antibacterial agents are as stated:
    (a) trimethoprim competitively inhibits the incorporation of para aminobenzoic acid (PABA) into dihydrofolic acid.
    (b) erythromycin blocks bacterial protein synthesis.
    (c) tetracyclines inhibit bacterial nucleic-acid synthesis.
    (d) ampicillin inhibits the formation of peptide cross-linkages during bacterial cell-wall synthesis.
    (e) chloramphenicol inhibits peptide-bond formation during bacterial protein synthesis.

144 The following statements are true:
    (a) sulphonamides can potentiate the action of tolbutamide.
    (b) sulphonamides are excreted more rapidly when the urine is rendered acidic.
    (c) sulphadimidine can be used to test acetylator status.
    (d) co-trimoxazole is a mixture of trimethoprim and sulphamethoxazole.
    (e) sulphonamides are secreted into breast milk

145 Benzylpenicillin:
    (a) can be effective when given orally to the very old.
    (b) excretion through the kidney is rapid in the neonate.
    (c) is usually injected.
    (d) excretion may be reduced by probenecid.
    (e) will not cause a hypersensitivity reaction in persons known to be hypersensitive to ampicillin.

142 (a) **True**
   (b) **True**   This route of administration, combined with its high lipid solubility, ensures a rapid onset of anaesthesia.
   (c) **False**   As thiopentone is very lipid soluble, it enters the highly perfused CNS rapidly, the anaesthetic action being terminated by redistribution from the CNS to other highly vascularized tissues. Metabolism does not account for its short duration of action.
   (d) **False**   No barbiturates have marked analgesic actions.
   (e) **False**   It has been used to control convulsions in status epilepticus and tetanus. In contrast, methohexitone (another intravenous short-acting barbiturate anaesthetic) frequently causes twitching, and occasionally convulsions.

143 (a) **False**   Sulphonamides inhibit the incorporation of PABA into dihydrofolic acid. Trimethoprim selectively inhibits bacterial dihydrofolate reductase which catalyses the reduction of dihydrofolic acid to tetrahydrofolic acid. A combination of trimethoprim and a sulphonamide (sulphamethoxazole) in the preparation co-trimoxazole provides a bactericidal mixture from two bacteristatic drugs.
   (b) **True**   Protein synthesis by bacterial ribosomes is inhibited without affecting human ribosomes.
   (c) **False**   Tetracyclines block bacterial protein synthesis. Tetracyclines accumulate in bacterial cells and achieve much higher concentrations there than in human cells and hence a selective antibacterial action is obtained. However, large doses can reduce protein synthesis in mammalian cells.
   (d) **True**   This leads to swelling and lysis of the cells.
   (e) **True**

144 (a) **True**   Some displacement of tolbutamide from plasma-binding sites may lead to an enhanced hypoglycaemic response.
   (b) **False**   Sulphonamides are weak acids. Rendering the urine acidic will decrease the degree of ionization and this will tend to reduce urinary excretion.
   (c) **True**   It is a relatively simple matter to measure the degree of acetylation of sulphadimidine in man. Acetylator status is considered important with regard to the metabolism and effects of several drugs, notably isoniazid, hydralazine and procainamide.
   (d) **True**
   (e) **True**   There is a small risk of kernicterus in jaundiced infants, particularly with long acting sulphonamides.

145 (a) **True**   Benzylpenicillin is inactivated by the action of acid in the stomach. Acid secretion in the elderly is reduced, so significant amounts of benzylpenicillin may be left available for absorption.
   (b) **False**   Penicillins are actively secreted into renal tubular fluid and such mechanisms are not fully developed in the neonate.
   (c) **True**
   (d) **True**   Probenecid blocks the active transport of penicillins into the kidney tubules, thus their excretion is reduced.
   (e) **False**   A person hypersensitive to one penicillin will be sensitive to other penicillins.

146 Chloramphenicol:
  (a) does not penetrate the blood-brain barrier.
  (b) must be administered parenterally.
  (c) can be safely used in premature infants.
  (d) can cause depression of bone marrow functions.
  (e) can cause discoloration of developing teeth when given to children.

146 (a) **False**
  (b) **False**   It is sufficiently lipid soluble to be given orally and to cross the blood-brain barrier.
  (c) **False**   It is highly toxic in neonates (particularly of low birth weight) in whom underdeveloped liver function does not allow adequate metabolism. It causes the 'grey syndrome', which is fatal in at least half of those affected.
  (d) **True**
  (e) **False**   Tetracyclines do this.

© 1991 A D'Mello and Z L Kruk

First published in Great Britain 1982.
Reprinted 1985
Second edition 1991

British Library Cataloguing in Publication Data

D'Mello, A.
  Multiple choice questions in pharmacology with
  answers and explanatory comments. – 2nd ed.
  I. Title   II. Kruk, Z. L.
  615.076

  ISBN 0-340-54321-3

Typeset in Helvetica Light by Hewer Text Compositions Services,
Edinburgh.
Printed and bound in Great Britain by Clays Ltd, St. Ives plc for
Edward Arnold, a division of Hodder and Stoughton Limited, Mill
Road, Dunton Green, Sevenoaks, Kent TN13 2YA.